314

Copyright @ 2017 Sue Regan Kenney

All rights reserved. No part of this book may be reproduced, stored in a retrieval system, or transmitted, in any form or by any means, without the prior written consent from the publisher and the author.

Published in 2017 by CreateSpace
www.createspace.com

Order information:
www.suekenney.ca
www.barebottomshoes.com

Cataloguing data available from Library and Archives Canada
ISBN-13: 978-1975719395
ISBN-10: 1975719395

Jacket design by Brian Foot
Book design/layout, copy editing by Joanne Haskins, thinkcom.ca

Cover photo from the author's collection.
Author photo by Deb Halbot

Disclaimer:
Any health-related information included in this book is not intended to substitute for qualified medical advice relevant to your individual case. All information is provided for educational purposes only. Please consult your doctor with questions or concerns before making any decisions about your health.

"Just like all of you, I was born a barefooter, but—for me at least—the years-long appeal of Chuck Taylors, Doc Martins and English-leather Oxfords made me all but forget the freedom of being naked from the ankles down. In her new book, Sue reminds us how much joy there is in releasing our inner child and tackling life with our toes and soles bared. And her stories inspire us to tread our own barefoot path to consciousness."
– Steve Lewis, MSc. BA. FRCGS; author, educator

"When Sue first showed up at my Toronto restaurant in bare feet in December I thought she had lost it. But she was so passionate about how good being barefoot made her feel and, besides the evidence in her earthy glow, the health benefits she raved about intrigued me.

I've always been a believer in the axiom 'You are what you eat,' which is why I feed people the healthiest food made by Mother Nature. I had never considered adding 'walking barefoot' to my health and wellness regimen of yoga, naps and organic plant food.

One day this past spring, while on my daily walk with my dog through Trinity Bellwoods Park, inspired by Sue, I slipped off my shoes and did the rest of my walk barefoot. It was a revelation for this urban heel-wearing concrete pounder.

I'm now an addict. It started slowly, tentatively, and over the course of the summer my tender little tootsies became more brave—pinecones and acorns don't hurt! I now purposely wear shoes that can be easily slipped on and off, and when I walk through the park I can't not take them off.

I have come to crave the sensuality of it: cool morning dew on tall blades of grass, a better stimulant than a cup of coffee; mid-afternoon sun-dried patches, radiating warmth like a heating pad on your soles; cushiony pineapple weed, nature's pillows.

My feet feel free! I feel alive and balanced, grounded and connected to the earth. If you're a skeptic like I was, read this and be inspired by Sue. Her passion for wearing bare feet is contagious."
– *Moira Nordholt, founder, Feel Good Guru*

"*Sue Kenney's passion for life is vivid and present in every page of* How to Wear Bare Feet. *If you ever wanted to get back to those carefree childhood days when it was a thrill to walk through the mud and grass with nothing between your toes and Mother Earth, this is the book for you. Sue is a natural guiding spirit, and she will walk you through it. Take off your shoes and socks and read this book!"*
– *Kevin Craig, barefooter and Author of* Burn Baby Burn Baby

"*As a personal trainer, developing sensory integration and health of the feet translates into a stronger body which provides proper locomotive biomechanics for human movement. As a barefooter I have never felt more balanced and in touch with myself as I do functioning barefoot. I want all my clients to feel the same. Sue's story is inspiring and will get you barefoot-ready."*
– *Meg McNeely, personal trainer/group fitness instructor*

How to Wear Bare Feet

by Sue Regan Kenney

Dedication

The stories in this book are offered in honor of the Great Mother Earth and to my dear Mum, who always encouraged me to play outside.

I dedicate this book to my daughters, Tara, Meghan and Simone and my grandchildren, Maeve, Laird, Jack, Heath and Nora, who constantly inspire me to remember my inner child.

Table of Contents

Acknowledgments ix
Author's Note xi
Foreword xvii
Introduction xxi

Chapter 1	A Bear Encounter 1
Chapter 2	The History of Shoes 5
Chapter 3	Sole to Soul 9
Chapter 4	Returning to the Mother Earth 13
Chapter 5	200,000 Sensory Receptors 15
Chapter 6	Facing Fear 19
Chapter 7	Germs and Stepping on Glass 21
Chapter 8	No Shoes. No Shirt. No Service. 25
Chapter 9	Barefoot Shoes 29
Chapter 10	Dr. Emily 33
Chapter 11	Sole Skin and Sweat 37
Chapter 12	Earthing 41
Chapter 13	Ecotherapy and Hydrotherapy 43
Chapter 14	Snow Bathing 47
Chapter 15	Anti-Aging and Movement Longevity 53
Chapter 16	Nutritional Mud 57
Chapter 17	Barefoot Babies 61
Chapter 18	Primal Running 65
Chapter 19	Barefoot on the Camino 67

Guide: How to Wear Bare Feet 73

Epilogue 79
Biography 82
Websites 83
Appendix 85
About the Author 93

Acknowledgments

I accord the highest honor and my eternal gratitude to the community of barefoot supporters around the world, whom I've encountered in person and on social media sites and who have inspired me with their stories and sage advice about embracing a barefoot lifestyle.

Immense gratitude goes to everyone who helped me to launch Barebottom Shoes, especially my dear mother, June Regan, and my daughters, Tara Kenney, Meghan Kenney-Elliott and Simone Kenney. I'm also immensely grateful to Luba Paolucci, Nancy O'Carroll, Marie Ostrowski, Jeannie Fast, Rod and Alejandra Romero, my Girlfriend Therapy Group, Steve Lewis, and, lastly, my sisters Pat Regan, Lorie Bos, Joanne Scott, Kelly Gibbs and my brother, Larry Regan, who backed my ideas and contributed many long hours to help me reach my dream.

Author's Note

My intention for writing *How to Wear Bare Feet* was based on the profound experiences I've had physically, mentally and spiritually, mostly as a result of walking barefoot in the forest. This was coupled with a personal desire to prove empirically that the body knows how to take care of itself naturally if we'd just get out of the way and let it.

The name of this book came out of a question people ask me all the time: "Where are your shoes?" I usually reply, "I'm wearing my bare feet!"

Do you remember the feeling of freedom and joy when you were a child running barefoot in the grass? On the last day of school, the first thing we did was kick off our shoes. Initially, the soles of our feet were tender, but within days we forgot all about it and we could run on gravel and pavement with ease.

When I reached the age of fifty-five I noticed there were numerous changes in my body that had compounded over time. In the morning, my entire body was stiff, regardless of whether I had been working out or doing yoga. In spring, fall and winter I was always cold, especially my hands and feet. Over the last twenty years I had developed flat arches, and my shoe size was half a size larger than in my thirties. The skin on the soles of my feet had become soft and extremely tender when I was without foot protection. Bunions were beginning to form on my left foot. My feet smelled all the time, and

I'd often get athlete's foot. I had calluses, cracks and severe dryness, too. I ground my teeth. My neck and back were sore or stiff most of the time. I had lousy posture. I was menopausal and had been diagnosed with vaginal atrophy, for which the doctor could suggest no cure other than topical estrogen cream or to try matcha. I also had asthma and was allergic to dogs and cats.

Around the same time I noticed that my legs were starting to bow outward, so my knees were no longer touching each other when I stood up, and this reminded me of my ninety-five-year-old grandmother, whom I adored. My hands were arthritic, and other joints seemed to be getting worse. I was a mess.

I'd always thought I would live to be 115, but my body was falling apart and I wasn't even half-way there. I had to do something radical, but I didn't know what. I didn't trust the medical profession to advise me on how to be healthier. The natural holistic industry had become so commercial it was hard to know what to believe anymore. I trusted my friend, Moira Nordholt, who owns Feel Good Guru in Toronto, and I ate anything she made and followed her advice. I did her raw vegan, organic cleanses; my digestive system thrived on this totally natural approach. The movement in my body was less than optimum. I had some degree of pain all the time.

Moira agreed with me that no one in our tribe was talking about what Mother Earth had to offer from the ground itself. What was in the mud and the dirt besides something for a face mask? Around this time there was a lot of talk about inflammation and an increase in autoimmune diseases. I was determined not to have to deal with any illness I could avoid. I began thinking about how our First Nations people had stayed so healthy. They wore moccasins with no support, slept on hides on the ground, used herbs for medicine, did ceremony and ate food foraged from the forest. Was something from the earth missing in our holistic approach to wellness?

From that place I researched barefooting and learned about earthing, human movement, foot function, anti-aging, footwear dangers, and why I was afraid of falling. It started with a paper by the 'Barefoot Professor,' Daniel Howell, PhD, titled "Foot Anatomy 101–Biofeedback." When I discovered how two hundred thousand neurotransmitter receptors in the soles of my feet were sending messages via a neural pathway to my brain about the terrain under my feet so they could work in harmony with my entire body to heal, protect, strengthen and set me on a new course of enlightenment, I was humbled.

Soon after, I started following Dr. Emily Splichal, a podiatrist in New York. She focused on sharing her knowledge about foot health, movement longevity and neuromuscular activation from the ground up and how these forces are transferred, and barefoot training. After I completed her Barefoot Training Specialist 1 course, my world changed forever.

My spiritual journey was kick-started in 2001 when I walked close to five hundred miles, alone in the winter, on the Camino de Santiago pilgrimage route in Spain. The thousand-year-old path traverses many forests and a variety of terrains on paths that encompass natural dirt, stone, pavement and concrete. During that journey I spent a great deal of time taking care of my feet and being aware of my boots in order to avoid blisters or injury so I could make it to the destination, Santiago. I walked for twenty-nine days and had a life-changing experience.

When I got home I continued obsessing over my feet—something I had more or less ignored most of my life except for getting the odd pedicure. Because of the Camino, the relationship I have with my feet is bonded to respect, gratitude and intimacy. It was clear to me they were absolutely committed to taking me wherever I asked them to go, and they were determined to keep me from harm.

An increase in consciousness and the new spiritual connection I had with Mother Earth because of walking intrigued me, and I started guiding other people on this mystical path. While walking I paid attention to the cadence of nature, the wisdom of the trees, the rhythm of the water, the magic of the wind, the mud in the earth, and the lessons of the seasons. She insisted I not be afraid of the animals, reptiles and insects but rather accept their medicine while listening closely to their guidance. Ultimately, this spiritual connection to her gave me strength, wisdom and love as I moved along the undulating forest floor. She taught me to trust my feet and embrace her world sole to soul. It's the perfect antidote to the damaging effects of civilization.

It's not a magic cream you can put on your feet, or a blanket you can sleep on, or a procedure that you can have someone else do for you. You have to take your shoes and socks off and put your bare feet on the ground and move. That's all. It's simple, it's free and it's accessible to anyone in the world. You don't have to be an athlete or be in great shape. But by doing it, I believe, every person can become stronger, healthier and more flexible, have better posture and be more balanced. Our feet are the foundation of our body, and they gift us with a direct connection to Mother Earth's infinite healing powers. When we wear shoes, the soles cut us off from nature and impede proper foot function.

I hesitated to begin my quest to share the benefits of barefooting, because I didn't have the credentials or academics to support calling myself a barefooting expert. Many people have encouraged me to write about my story. I've been training my body for various sports and dance, or coaching sports, my entire life. Several years ago I was part of a crew of women who won the FISA World Rowing Masters Regatta. I'm a Level 2 rowing coach, I studied reflexology and Reiki, and I completed five ten-day silent Vipassana meditation retreats in India, Canada and Spain.

It's been almost seven years since I first put my bare soles on the ground to go for a walk. I'm now sixty-one with three daughters and five grandchildren. In that time I've experienced numerous health advantages, anti-aging benefits, a connection to nature that was unprecedented in my life, improvements in posture and alignment, and a keen understanding of how my brain responds to the sensory feedback it obtains from soles of my feet.

If you intuitively feel drawn to being connected to the earth as an imperative to good health, then this book will help support your decision from a common-sense point of view. In this book I share stories with you about my personal re-wilding journey, my gathering of empirical evidence about the benefits of embracing a barefoot lifestyle while living in a cottage near the forest on the shores of Lake Couchiching. For those of you who want to return to a more natural state—physically, mentally and spiritually—barefooting is an excellent mindfulness practice as well as a whole-body health and movement practice.

You'll be given a guide on how to create a daily practice to 'wear' bare feet at the end of the book, along with some resources you can investigate to support this ideology.

Are you ready to take the first step? Here it is: take your shoes off while you are reading this, so you can personally experience the book from the perspective of the soles of your feet. It's your human right.

Foreword

Spirituality and Barefooting

I met Sue Regan Kenney in 2009 at a local market in Muskoka, Ontario, where she was busy sharing stories and promoting her book, My Camino, from which she earned the status of best-selling author. We became instant friends from that very first meeting. The similarities of our lives were uncanny. We discovered we both came from large traditional "religious" families, each with seven children—six girls and one boy—and both of us the second child and born in the same year. Little did either of us know then what life moving forward would reveal through us on our journey to self-love and inner awakening. Looking back eight years now, both of our paths are so obvious and the support of friendship clearly no accident. Our respective experiences have shown that it takes tremendous persistence to continue the unconventional journey to reveal our inner potential, enlightenment, and to step out of our comfort zone of fitting in. It is true that we don't always understand life moving forward but, looking back, it all makes perfect sense. Neither of us then could have guessed our respective paths as they revealed themselves over time.

After hearing about Sue's many experiences on the Camino de Santiago, I decided to walk the Camino myself from St Jean Pied de Port in France to Finisterre in its entirety. There are no words to describe this journey, mile after mile of walking alongside the sounds of one's own silence, breath and inner thoughts. Yes, the experiences on this path throughout are completely in sync and supportive of an organic spiritual awakening. I could totally relate to Sue's earlier experiences walking the Camino and this path, which was all for her and her life's work and, as she was called to take her shoes off, for her to bare the soles of her feet and connect to Mother Earth. Why was this so necessary? As Sue discovered, it was so the energy between her physical body and the earth's body could entangle through the neural pathways of the feet that connect to her brain and rewire her organic body to its fullest conscious expression of oneness with all life. After all, it is through our brain that we are able to access multiple dimensions of the universe. Never discount that our feet and brain are in constant communication.

And so it was that in 2012 our respective journeys toward enlightenment and self-love began. Sue chose to be barefoot at home in Muskoka, which is known for its unspoiled beauty, lakes and natural habitats abundant in wildlife. I made the choice to go to India to study spirituality and science and experience the different dimensions and states of consciousness. My guru and teacher is a Poonar Avatar, an incarnation who by his very presence heals and aligns a person through shaktipada: entanglement with his state-space to its highest potential, experiencing the state of Oneness. What I am sharing here may sound extreme in conjunction with the old paradigm and belief system, especially the religious route many of us grew up in and around, which has us participating in the effects of what life dishes out. This creates victim mentality that is fear-based and not a spiritual truth.

Science, quantum physics and metaphysics have been revealing more truth-quantifying energy, specifically the Kundalini energy as the spiritual foundation for awakening. Kundalini is our inner potential energy lying dormant at the base of our spine simply because we have lost sight of our true nature. Our negative views about emotions, our attachments and we ourselves have twisted our passage of Kundalini.

We have become afraid to live powerfully and with confidence. Without continuous validation from others we are almost afraid of who we are. Let's face it; many of us carry a lot of guilt. Consider this guidance from Om Shanti: "When our scale of consciousness is no longer limited to our body but envelops the whole universe, kundalini becomes a power source when it reaches the crown chakra, breaking free of the shackles of thoughts, desires, emotions, and instead our commands manifest a new reality as the fears and conditioning dwindle and a new paradigm, becoming the master of our own universe, dawns like the sun on a new day."

I remember when my guru said recently that it was good to go barefoot. Bare feet are common at the ashram in India, and shoes are not worn inside. I was so excited to share this with Sue, as all the research she has done speaks to the nerve-endings and connections on the bottom of our feet that awaken whole-brain activity, which she shares with you in this book. The facts are accurate and truthful. A truth is something that has to be experienced. Sue shares her barefoot experiences on her journey and shares the miraculous effects on our whole being. Whenever I return from India, I share with Sue the spiritual exercises we practiced and what expansion and experiences were had. Invariably, she is going through something equally as profound.

Lastly, I would like to bring awareness and attention to the awakening of the third eye, because it is one of the most important processes for raising consciousness. Experiencing the inner space happens through the third eye, as it reflects our outer conditions. It

Sue Regan Kenney

is from this inner world contained in the browsing center that our outer world reflects back to us. As noted in Matthew 6:22, "The light of the body is the eye: if therefore thine eye be single, thy whole body shall be full of light." The eye pertains to inner consciousness because everything is inner consciousness. Sue shared with me her profound experience of seeing the luminai naturai, the light of nature, within the Amazon jungles of Ecuador.

This is a book full of timely information on how to heal our bodies, be physically powerful in our lives, reclaim our mental health and live authentically with integrity as an expression and contribution for the well-being of all.

Be curious, open your hearts, raise your self, and listen.

— HrNr Ma Nithya Muktiroopananda (Nancy O'Carroll)
Healer and spiritual teacher

Introduction

Gone are the days of viral debates and forums on the benefits versus the risks of barefoot running. Newspapers such as *The New York Times* have shifted their focus away from discrediting minimal footwear companies, and the "Vibram lawsuit" is old news. As the dust settles on the barefoot-running debate, we must ask ourselves: Did the benefits of barefooting actually exist? Or was all of this barefoot talk just a fad?

As a podiatrist, human-movement specialist and creator of the Barefoot Training Specialist® Certification, I can confidently say no! The power of foot and barefoot science is far from a fad. Sure, perhaps five-fingered footwear was a fad, but the science of plantar proprioception and the integrated human foot… that, my friend, is not a fad.

Since 2010 I've been dedicating my podiatry career to changing the way patients and professionals around the world think about footwear, barefoot science and what I call foot-to-core sequencing. Through my education company, EBFA Global, I've been able to travel across the globe introducing foot medicine and barefoot training to countries in which formal podiatry doesn't exist. From China and India to Norway and Portugal, people of all ages are beginning to embrace the true power of being barefoot.

Experts such as Sue have played a critical role in changing the perception around a barefoot lifestyle. Through her dedication to the art of earthing and teaching others how to reconnect body, mind and sole to the ground we move on, countless lives have been affected.

Back when I first started lecturing on barefoot science, my focus was primarily on the direct stimulation of the skin on the bottom of the feet and its role in balance training for seniors. It's funny when I look back at my old presentations and how I wasn't even scraping the surface as to how powerful the foot is in movement and performance!

The pivotal step in the evolution of Barefoot Strong was when I left my surgical residency training to go back to graduate school and get my Master's in Human Movement. To leave a medical residency in the middle of training was a decision that could have cost me the ability to ever practice medicine. Despite this risk, in my heart I knew I needed to take this step. My intuition was telling me that I needed to connect the dots in my knowledge and perspective on the foot and human movement. I knew that there was more to this barefoot concept than simply balance training and proprioception.

The next two years were dedicated to the exploration of human movement as it relates to the foot, barefoot science and the fascial integration between the feet and core. The research I uncovered took my podiatric medical degree to a level I never dreamed possible. With this new in-depth knowledge of foot-to-core fascial integration, neuromuscular coordination and small-nerve proprioception, I knew I was onto something powerful.

What I discovered was that the biggest secret when it comes to being barefoot. To truly be Barefoot Strong you must be barefoot *with a purpose*—Intentional Foot Activation.

In the human body we have 206 muscles, all of which are surrounded by a special type of tissue called fascia. Perhaps you've heard of foam rolling or have seen ads for a trendy new product called the

How to Wear Bare Feet

Fascia Blaster. Whatever your association with fascia may be thus far, we can think of fascia as a type of Saran Wrap that connects every muscle in the body to each other. It is this web-like connection of our muscles that allows the feet to influence the upper leg and hip or allows the dexterity of the hand to influence the stability of the shoulder blade.

In fact, it is this fascia that connects the muscles of the feet to the muscles of the deep core or pelvic floor, establishing what's called the foot-to-core connection. This is fascial connection as known as our Deep Front Fascial Line and is based on a book called *Anatomy Trains* by Thomas Myers. If we want to take this one step further, not only does fascia connect our feet to our pelvic floor, but fascia also connects our pelvic floor to our diaphragm. This means that core stability is connected to the way we breathe, and that the way we breathe can, theoretically, impact foot stability.

We can activate and connect into this Deep Front Line via an exercise called Short Foot. You can find many videos on YouTube about how to perform short-foot exercises; however, if you are looking to take this exercise to the next level I recommend coordinating your breathing with this exercise. To activate the body's foot-to-core pathway I suggest performing short-foot exercise while exhaling and engaging the pelvic floor. To learn more, please visit www.youtube.com/ebfafitness.

Regardless of our country, religion or educational background, there is a unified connection between us all, a connection between the foot and the world we live on. To be Barefoot Strong is more than to simply work out or running without shoes.

Barefoot Strong is a lifestyle. It does not mean simply going about your day not wearing shoes; rather, there is an appreciation for the ground on which we move. To be Barefoot Strong there is an appreciation of impact forces and the valuable information that enters the foot with every step we take. To be Barefoot Strong there is an appreciation of the neuromuscular system and how our foot connects to the core, creating reflexive stability. To be Barefoot Strong there is an appreciation of the earth and the ground on which our ancestors evolved.

Are you ready to embark on this journey with me? It's time to get Barefoot Strong!

— Dr. Emily Splichal, DPM, MS, CES
Functional podiatrist and movement specialist, creator Barefoot Training Specialist® Certification, author *Barefoot Strong | Unlock the Secret to Movement Longevity*

Chapter 1

A Bear Encounter

My plan was to write the first-draft manuscript for this book as my project for the Muskoka Novel Marathon event. This is not a running event but, rather, a fund-raiser for an area literacy foundation. Forty writers get together for three days in mid-July. They get sponsors to donate to the cause, and they inspire each other to write for seventy-two hours straight. I had done this writing marathon before and found it to be a great way to get motivated and get my first draft down on paper.

The night before the event, I bought a sign that read "Bear Feet Always Welcome." Made of metal, it profiled a black bear. It would be fun to see it on my desk as I wrote barefoot the entire weekend. I packed up the sign, my laptop, a sleeping bag, my favorite coffee mug and a few other things I would need for the weekend and loaded them into the car.

On my way to the event I stopped at my favorite hiking trail, Kahshe Barrens. The wooded property winds through a natural dirt trail almost four miles long; I love to walk or run barefoot on it at least a couple of times a week. I wrote my first book after a five-hundred-mile walk, and I believed there was a relationship between walking and creativity. It seemed fitting to walk this trail before I started writing again.

About ten minutes into my walk, it became obvious my pace could not remain leisurely. Deer flies and mosquitoes were feasting on me. Being barefoot didn't stop me from running, so I picked up speed to try to outpace them. As I navigated the rolling path through the forest, I shot a short video about running in nature with my cell phone to share with people on social media. Every so often I stopped and bent down low to the ground to see if the bugs would keep flying past over my head, but, when I stood up, they were right there ready to attack.

After the first loop of almost two miles, I was still being eaten alive. I had bites all over, and my arms were completely covered with mosquitoes, black flies and deer flies. I stopped to take a picture to share with the other writers, but before I could press the button, I heard something move in front of me. It sounded heavy and moved slow. I stayed still and scanned the forest. Again, something moved in the bushes. Looking in the direction of the noise, I squinted my eyes a couple of times to confirm what I thought I was seeing: a real, live Canadian black bear. It was standing only thirty feet away, and it was obviously much bigger than a cub. It made a huffing noise and looked directly at me. The hair on my arms stood on end. I was scared.

The common advice about encounters with a black bear is to raise one's hands in the air to appear taller and to stand one's ground confidently. Easy to say—tricky to do as I stood there, aware of how vulnerable I was. We made eye contact and I was awestruck, but at the same time I couldn't help but wonder if it was a female or a male. It lifted one of its huge paws off the ground and stretched it toward me. I wanted to run. I became very stiff as a chill ran through my body. Now I knew I was in a very serious situation.

Almost instinctively I jerked my arms up into the air to make myself bigger, and then I growled back at it with the deepest voice I could muster out of my fear. Nothing happened. I longed to communicate with the bear that I was not interested in harming it or its cubs—if there were any—and that I desperately wanted to send it love. The bear made that huffing noise again, and I wanted to run.

Once again I thought of all the advice I'd been given. Every piece of literature I'd ever read and every person I spoke to said not to run. I wondered if any of these experts had been standing thirty feet from a bear that was looking straight at them at the time and been wearing only running shorts and a singlet, barefoot, waiting to see who was going to move first. Since the bear wasn't moving, I knew I had to make a decision.

I cautiously turned half way to the side and slowly shuffled toward a tree, thinking maybe I could hide behind it. The bear huffed at me and slammed its paw on the ground. Very slowly I stepped backward, keeping my eye on the bear, which seemed to be moving back onto its haunches. The trail was narrow, covered with tree roots and rocks that would have made it very difficult to maneuver in reverse if I had been in shoes. Fortunately, I could feel every bump and change in terrain on the soles of my feet, and I adapted immediately to the shifting environment. This gave me a sense of confidence. I growled a friendly growl, as if to say goodbye, and awkwardly ran away holding my arms up in the air. Against my better judgment I had taken my eye off the bear, and now I didn't want to look back.

I heard rustling again in the bushes, and the huffing sound was getting closer. The bear was following me. I imagined myself lying on my back on the forest floor as an easy target, the bear running toward me, digging his claws into me. Had I make a huge mistake? Was I now going to be attacked by the bear? I almost wished I'd taken a picture so at least my family could piece together how I was mauled to death. For a split second I felt disappointment with myself: if I died now, I wouldn't have the chance to write this book; I regretted not writing it sooner.

My running form was quiet and swift with a gentle landing. By lifting my knees as high as I could, I was confident I wouldn't trip on a root or a rock. The rustling seemed to get louder. I felt my breath laboring; all the blood in my arms had drained. I was running so fast the deer flies couldn't catch up. Moments later, the thump of the bear's footsteps faded and the squirrels became curious again. Everything around me was still. The birds were chirping and the bear was gone. Life in the forest went back to the natural order. My encounter with the bear seemed dreamlike, almost as though it had never happened.

After about a mile I finally reached the end of the loop, which meant I was about another mile from the safety of the parking lot. Once I was safe, it was easier to be grateful for the chance to connect with a bear in its own habitat without being attacked. It was a perfect barefoot encounter.

When I reached the Muskoka Novel narathon site, I looked up Ted Andrew's book *Animal Speaks* and searched for "Bear totem" and what medicine it represents. I found out Bear is a spirit animal that is in touch with the cycles of nature and the trees. When Bear shows up in your life, it's time to stand for your beliefs and your truth. It symbolizes warrior spirit and the courage to fight. Its medicine is also related to introspection and healing.

It was Bear medicine that set me up to write this book. I could now hold up my arms in declaration of my intention to speak from my authentic self and share my vision of a barefoot movement. What I was to learn next changed the course of my life and confirmed this was the right barefoot path.

Chapter 2

The History of Shoes

The most common shoe for thousands of years was the moccasin, which is still worn today. We think the oldest shoes made of leather were found on the Ice Man, who lived over 5,500 years ago. Records show other shoes made of sage are up to ten thousand years old, and animal-skin boots were worn up to fifty-five thousand years ago to protect feet from freezing weather and snow. Since the skins were precious, footwear was reserved for when it was absolutely needed, such as in a life-threatening situation. The world's oldest known shoes are sagebrush sandals. They are about ten thousand years old and were found in Fort Rock, Oregon.[1]

You can learn a lot about a culture based on its footwear. The history of footwear represents the development of a class structure for most societies. Before the industrial revolution, shoes were expensive and were worn for years and often passed down. The pump (worn by both men and women) and the Oxford shoe were designed in fifteenth-century England, changing the history of shoes forever.

Selecting footwear today can require a lot of thought; people know they will be judged on the quality and condition of their shoes. For

---

[1] University of Oregon Museum of Natural and Cultural History, http://natural-history.uoregon.edu/shoes02

many, shoes signal social class and status, and it can affect the way we are treated in our communities, public places, stores and restaurants.

Women have been told since they were young girls that they must wear heels to enhance their attractiveness and sexuality. They choose high-heeled shoes usually based on design, not comfort or fit. Why should women feel they must look good in footwear that ultimately deforms their feet and affects the rest of their body too? More recently, many celebrities, including Julia Roberts, have gone barefoot to make a statement at red-carpet events whose dress code requires women to wear high heels.

In the 1970s it was understood that athletic shoes needed to have extra padding, that any kind of pronation of the foot wasn't good and, therefore, we had to buy shoes that would help correct that fault. Because we were led to believe that a heel strike would help to propel the foot forward, rocking it onto the toe for the push-off, more padding was desired. We all bought the shoes and paid dearly for them. Their stiff soles didn't allow the foot or toes to move, again wreaking havoc with foot function. We jammed our heels so hard that it caused more injuries. Little did we know as teenagers that these shoes would deform our feet to the point where we would have trouble walking and balancing in everyday situations as we aged. Forty years later, we were informed that the running shoes we'd been wearing all our lives were now damaging for our feet and body.

Katy Bowman, author of *Whole Body Barefoot*, is a biomechanist by training andtrains people on alignment and load-science. She explains in clear, science-based terms the issues created by conventional shoes. She describes in detail the steps necessary to transition to more natural footwear.

How to Wear Bare Feet

> In general, conventional footwear is narrower than the foot in its unshod state, has an elevated heel, and is stiff and thick-soled. Shoes can press the toes together, which weakens the foot musculature, thereby affecting nerve health. Elevated heels make it impossible to access the full range of motion of many joints – which in turn creates highly repetitive but small motions in the hips and knees. And because all your parts are connected, you have to make constant adjustments to the pelvis and spine in order to stay upright, while you're essentially walking downhill (your toes are below your ankles, thanks to your heeled shoes) on flat ground.

In her book she reminds us there are twenty-six bones, thirty-three joints, nineteen muscles and 107 ligaments in your feet. Focusing on strengthening your feet will correct your body's alignment. By wearing shoes with less support you will create more reliance on the function of your foot's tendons and muscles, and that makes you stronger. The more supportive the footwear, the less the foot has to do; the muscles will atrophy.

What I learned from Bowman is that as long as you have a heel on your shoe, even on men's shoes or on ballet flats, your body is out of alignment. To experience this, I stood up and, keeping my feet slightly apart, I imagined wearing shoes with a very low heel. By lifting my heel about half an inch off the floor to notice what my body does, I could tell I was leaning forward slightly. My belly was soft.

Try it. Is your neck protruding? Are you balanced? Drop your heels to the floor and be aware about how that lift affects your posture. Try it again, only this time imagine you're wearing heels that are about two inches high and notice how stressed your body is. Do your core muscles engage? For me, it was like I was leaning slightly backward. Is your posture upright? Do you feel more balanced and grounded? After this simple exercise, it made sense to me that our feet should rest even with the floor.

The soles of our feet were designed to balance us when we aren't wearing shoes. Because I was covering the soles of my feet, they couldn't do their job. Utilizing my body's intelligence from the feet up was the answer to my health dilemma.

Chapter 3

Sole to Soul

When I began leading groups on the Camino pilgrimage, one thing that was clear to me each time I came home, year after year, was that in order to live my purpose, to use my voice to inspire people on their life journey to return to their authentic self, I had to keep walking. So I walked in the city, in parks and on the beach. I especially loved walking in the forest in Muskoka near my cottage, wearing high-tech Italian leather boots with thick soles and stiff ankles. Throughout those years, I worked on several highly creative projects, and I walked religiously. Walking helped keep my mind at peace, inspired creativity, kept me on the Camino back home.

My decision to leave Toronto was partly because my children had all moved away. It was also because it had just become too noisy for me. Longing for a more simple life, I moved to my little cottage on Lake Couchiching, closer to nature.

One day after a walk in the forest, I felt a calling to be still. I decided to meditate and went down to the waterfront to sit on the huge granite rock that skirted the shore. I took off my boots and socks, setting the soles of my feet on the rugged Precambrian shield of granite that covered the land, and I was at peace.

Without warning, an energetic charge ran through my feet and up my body, like a sonic burst of Kundalini energy traveling through each of the seven chakras and released through my crown. The residue of its path was evident as all the sensory nerve endings on the soles of my feet tingled. It tickled the skin on my arms; it raised goose bumps on my legs and made my blood rush faster and my heart beat stronger. I smiled from ear to ear as I understood exactly what I was meant to do.

Looking up to the sky in gratitude, I chuckled in a way reminiscent of the laughing Buddha. It was absolutely clear to me that I should be barefoot.

Immediately I got up and walked on the granite, and then I walked slowly on the grass, experiencing the cool, damp sensation on my feet. In a couple of minutes I had walked to my driveway, which was covered with limestone gravel. I hesitated to put my bare feet on the stones.

The first step sent me into shock as pain surged into the delicate soles of my feet. My back hunched forward and my knees bent to relieve the weight. Stepping again, as gently as I could while spreading the weight over the balls of my feet, I made odd groaning noises and tried to focus on my breath to ease the pain. It still hurt. I was already convinced this was not something I wanted to do. It was just too painful.

Yet the day after, I went back outside on the grass. I decided to make it a daily practice with the intention to walk barefoot until I didn't feel pain—trying to think of it as a sensation, not good or bad. For several weeks while I walked, the soles of my feet responded to the sensation of the limestone with tension and disdain. The only way I could approach those sharp rocks was to focus on my breath and not look down. If I saw the gravel, I would perceive my experience to be more painful than what I was really feeling.

How to Wear Bare Feet

Eventually I made it to the gravel-covered road and started to walk down it. Many people in the neighborhood asked me why I would attempt to walk barefoot on the road when it hurt so much. I explained my commitment to being more connected to the earth. I truly believed I could overcome the pain, and in time I did.

Chapter 4

Returning to Mother Earth

Going barefoot was an experience I didn't expect to be spiritual, enlightening and fun, too. My soul was calling me to return to a more natural, even tribal, way of living.

I walked in the forest barefoot several times a week, and I covered 140 miles each time on the Camino, twice a year. I developed a deep love and connection with Mother Earth. Whenever I spent time in the forest I felt extremely happy, content and full of energy. When I stayed away from its energy, I felt lonely. It made me wonder why that was happening.

One day I came home from a barefoot walk with another clear message that I should guide people back to the forest. It was obvious to me that once they were in nature she would take care of them. This spurred the idea to post comments and photos on social media of me in my bare feet to introduce people to walking in the forest. In the narration they were encouraged to go barefoot, touch the trees and the earth, feel the rocks, step in the mud and streams and even drink the spring water if they were so inclined. People loved it, and that encouraged me to keep going.

When walking I found myself longing to touch the trees and leaves with my hands at the same time the soles of my feet were touching the forest floor. Sometimes I would lie down on the forest floor and look up at the trees and sky. The forest was my playground. A profound connection to my inner child was activated when I started climbing trees, something I hadn't done since I was a kid. By experiencing nature from a whole-body perspective, I engaged in a deeper sense of closeness to my body and to the world around me. There, I was rediscovering my inner child, and I liked her.

Our ancestors went barefoot in all kinds of weather and on varying terrain. They wore their moccasins only in extreme conditions because the animal skins were so precious; they needed them to last for years. It is now reversed. We wear our shoes in all conditions because they are so precious, and yet our bare feet can outlast them by a lifetime. Do we have our priorities in the right order?

Chapter 5

200,000 Sensory Receptors

When I finally got used to walking on gravel, the sensation of pain was virtually gone. Now my feet longed for the stimulation of gravel or stones on my soles. It was like natural reflexology.

There was a sense of freedom and joy as I moved through the woods. It took some time to adjust to a mid-strike barefoot gait. At times the skin on my soles would split open, and that was quite painful. On one of the barefoot social media pages, I learned that Crazy Glue was a perfect remedy, since it was invented to bind skin together in place of stitches, and it worked.

At first I was constantly stubbing my toes because they were too weak to lift up during my gait, likely from wearing shoes so much in the past. In shoes, our toes lie mostly flat on the sole and the shoe does the work. Like all muscles in the body, if they aren't used they will atrophy. Imagine hiking boots as a soft cast for the foot. If you've ever broken a bone, you know that after six weeks in a cast all the muscles have atrophied and you must do physiotherapy to strengthen them again. Think of the shape of the muscles in your feet after they've been in shoes and boots for thirty, forty or fifty years.

When I started barefooting in the city, I wasn't sure how safe it was, and I wasn't that comfortable in public without shoes on. (I'll talk more about practical barefooting later in the book.) When barefoot, I tried to walk more lightly and not pound my heels into the ground, as I had become accustomed to doing in shoes. Someone posted a link to a blog about biofeedback from the soles of our feet to help monitor and fine-tune the proper mechanics of walking and running. Having never heard of this, I was curious.

It was written by the 'Barefoot Professor,' Daniel Howell, PhD, author of *The Barefoot Book*. "Foot Anatomy 101 – Biofeedback" was one page of text that rocked my world. It gave me the courage to continue barefooting with a new understanding about how exposing my feet to the ground could help my brain gather information.

After reading the article, I was even more anxious to expand my experimental learning, and I fully committed to honoring the sensory receptors in the soles of my feet and their relationship with my central nervous system. I found out about natural biofeedback as it relates to the mechanics of walking and running. The paper is so important that I share it in its entirety in the Appendix.

This information changed the way I thought about barefooting. It was no longer only about a connection to the earth; it was the solution to movement longevity and self-healing. The function of the sensory nerve receptors is to experience and record every detail about the surface and area around the foot and then store this data in the brain so the body responds efficiently and effectively, making subtle adjustments in the bones and joints. It was impossible for me to ignore the negative impact of wearing shoes all the time. It was time to let go of all the fears about barefooting and give my body a chance to do what it knew best. In all the sports, walking, courses and workshops I have done in my life, never had the importance of bare soles been mentioned. I have to wonder why this information is being withheld from us.

How to Wear Bare Feet

When we spend a lifetime in soled footwear, it's easy to commit to investing time to retrain the sensory nerve receptors to take in this information. I see it like teaching Siri how to pronounce words or names you use. Once she is given a noun she doesn't quite understand, she asks for clarification. Your feet are like the keyboard for your brain. The more senses, temperatures and experiences you type into the soles, the bigger the vocabulary it has to communicate to the brain and the central nervous system, and they will ultimately adapt every organ and body system.

Related to this topic is neuroplasticity. In the book *The Brain That Changes Itself*, author Norman Doidge talks about how neural pathways adapt to their usage. The body works on an energy quota and is always trying to be more efficient. Neural pathways take up energy to manage. If after some time the data that is being routed from your body to your brain is no longer being sent, the brain will disconnect that pathway to conserve energy.

For example, if you keep wearing closed-in shoes with soles, the message being sent is that it is hot, flat and sweaty inside your shoes; there is no message about the actual temperature, the environment or terrain and other feedback. Therefore, the central nervous system needs to adapt only a few systems in your body to manage the 'wrong' environment. You will need to put a sweater on, extra socks, slippers and maybe even a scarf. If the same message is sent repeatedly, the neural pathway will identify this as wasted energy and cut it off.

The good news is that the brain is forgiving and will re-establish new pathways when required. It's still possible to re-introduce sensations to the two hundred thousand exteroceptors in the soles of your feet. You can start right now and at the same time exercise your brain!

Today I am rarely ever too hot or too cold. The receptors respond in milliseconds to changes in the ground. By relaying this information efficiently to all the systems in my body, they adjust with ease to keep me safe and healthy. My feet slowly adapted to the external environment of pavement and concrete through practice.

Believe it or not, there are even more benefits. I was about to meet the podiatrist I mentioned earlier, Dr. Emily Splichal, who would teach me about impact forces, fascial fitness and foot-to-core sequencing.

First, let's talk about some of the fears around practical barefooting.

Chapter 6

Facing Fear

Our feet are one of the most intimate parts of our body and, when exposed, they can free us of our inhibitions. Barefooting can be liberating for the body and the mind. Many years ago I signed up for a theater arts class that took place on the stage in the auditorium. On the first day, our teacher asked us to sit in a circle with our legs stretched out and our feet pointed toward the middle. Then he told us to take off our shoes and socks. We complained—what was the point of doing that?—and giggled awkwardly.

Then he told us how our feet can be intimate. When we expose our bare feet, we reveal an innermost aspect of ourselves. As actors, he wanted us to let down our guard to be free to express our authentic self through our characters and roles. If we could stand on stage and deliver our lines in our bare feet, he assured us, we would be grounded and confident. It was at that moment in my life I realized there was a part of myself I hadn't revealed to the world.

We each took turns reading a piece alone on stage, and it was mesmerizing to watch as each student delivered from their soul. That day our teacher gave us a life tool for facing fear. It also gave me permission to reveal myself publicly, in my bare feet. Sadly, I had forgotten this life skill until I started giving keynote talks in my bare feet. I've never felt so incredibly grounded on stage.

Sue Regan Kenney

When I started barefooting, I was afraid of being judged by my family and friends. Would I be asked to leave a store or restaurant? Would I get bitten by a snake or step on dog poop? Would I ever get a date again? Each time I stepped out of the house in my bare feet was an opportunity for me to face a fear. It also gave me practice in letting go of the judgment of others—it was their stuff, not mine.

Most people think that in order to go barefoot, it's mind over matter, that you must have tough feet to withstand the pain, like you do when walking on hot coals. That's just not so. I personally would never walk on hot coals, because I could burn the soles of my feet, but after some practice I can now walk on snow!

Chapter 7

Germs and Stepping on Glass

You don't have to be subversive to be a barefooter.

When we think of germs, we assume we are protected from them because of our shoes. When was the last time you washed the inside of your shoes? Bacteria live and thrive in moisture and heat, and that means the inside of your shoes or boots is a perfect environment for them to breed. When you take your shoes off to go into someone's home, you are actually leaving that bacteria throughout the house.

When we walk barefoot, we constantly exfoliate the soles of our feet. If by chance we do step on something with germs, there's a good possibility we will brush it off on the ground or in the grass during the following steps we take. By exposing our soles to different bacteria, the body builds up resistance, but when our feet are always inside shoes, there is no exposure and the skin becomes soft and weak.

Of course many big cities have exceptionally dirty streets and we have to be careful about where we walk. When I first tried barefooting in the city I was reminded of what my mother told me about bacteria on cloth baby diapers. She said to make sure I put them outside on the clothesline to dry, because the sun bleached them and in the process killed all the bacteria.

To avoid germs when barefooting in a city, I usually walk on the sunny side of the street because the sun kills bacteria. After it rains, the streets are definitely cleaner. If you're not sure about the sidewalks, wear shoes and, regardless of the environment, always wash your feet as soon as you get home.

Several years ago I visited India for three months to study Vipassana meditation. I traveled from Delhi to Jaipur and Mumbai to Kutch in the north, often visiting small villages. There were one billion people in the country, and I was curious to see how they approached hygiene practices with other people. They shared water bottles and water cups, but their lips never touched the rims when they drank because of the way they poured the water into their mouths. This saved on buying extra water bottles: they could buy a large one for several people.

They squatted over a hole instead of sitting on a toilet seat and rarely used toilet paper. They never kissed strangers or shook their hands; instead they put their own hands in a prayer position and while bowing forward would say, "Namaste," which means, "I honor the light within you."

Adults and kids walk all over India barefoot and they never worry about it. They don't have fear or see the harm in doing it. One day in Varanasi it rained, and I was in sandals. I couldn't avoid stepping into the cow manure, because it mixed with the rainwater and turned into mud. It was so gross at first, but everyone was doing it. It seemed that whatever germs they picked up helped to build antibodies, so they could fight disease without prescriptions, since many couldn't afford them anyway.

When I hear about Tom's Shoes giving away a free pair of shoes to kids in Third World countries, I'm disappointed. The bigger problem there is not being barefoot, but rather not having clean water to drink and a place to sleep with a roof overhead. They are marketing to a young audience who will potentially one day make enough money to buy a pair of branded shoes. Just because we have ruined our feet and diminished our health by wearing shoes all the time, it shouldn't be encouraged in Third World countries for profit. If you think of it, we were born barefoot, and the majority of the world's population is barefoot most of the time.

The first major fear for most people when they see a barefooter is the danger of stepping on glass. When I started barefooting I was always looking where I was going. If I saw something dangerous, I walked around it or jumped over it. For obvious reasons, I avoid going barefoot where groups have been partying and breaking beer bottles in a park.

In shoes we have the tendency to slide our feet along. There is no fear of getting cut or stubbing your toes, because they are protected. When I walk barefoot, I tend to lift my feet up with each step and pay attention to the ground. If there is a sharp piece of glass sticking up out of the ground, you could cut your foot, but rarely do you find that situation. The best advice is to be cautious.

Our body is designed to take care of itself. Take your shoes and socks off and give your feet a chance.

Chapter 8

No Shoes. No Shirt. No Service.

Someone once said to me that the opposite of courage is conformity.

Sadly, numerous social barriers prevent people from going barefoot in the city, despite the incredible benefits. Shoes are now taken for granted in every situation. Barefooters are often judged and put into categories that don't present as valuable to society: hippies, the poor, the mentally ill, homeless people, artists, the unemployed, and more. That's not a fair judgment of those individuals or of barefooters.

More often than not, barefooters desire to be connected to nature, and some are even on a mission to reduce their environmental footprint. They are compassionate, courageous individuals who care about their health and want to be free to make choices about their footwear.

Back in the 1960s many stores put up signs that said *No Shoes. No Shirt. No Service.* They were directed at males with long hair who were shirtless. Since women didn't usually wear shirts—they wore blouses or other tops—or go topless in public, that seemed obvious. The shopkeepers wanted to keep these males out of their stores because of the way they looked. Strangely, this sign seemed to work.

One day I finished my walk in the forest and went to a large grocery store in town. I preferred doing business in local shops, but my daughters and their families were coming for the weekend and I needed to buy bigger quantities. Feeling a bit lost in the huge space,

I pushed the buggy around slowly as I searched the long aisles for what I needed.

Two men in store uniforms approached me. One man introduced himself as the manager of the store. The other man stood behind him looking at the floor. He asked me if I had any shoes with me, and I replied, "I'm wearing my bare feet." He was not amused and told me the health code prevented me from shopping in their store shoeless. I asked, "What health code?" He couldn't answer and only repeated that I had to leave. I suggested that I needed to pick up some more things and I wouldn't be long. I promised not to touch anything, except the floor, with my feet. He assured me that wouldn't be possible and I had to leave the store right away or they would have to call the police. The other man stepped forward and stood by his side, ready to take action if I were going to be difficult.

Honestly, I was more embarrassed and humiliated by them than anything. I turned on my bare heel and, leaving my buggy where it was, walked out of the store feeling frustrated. They followed me right to the door. I ran to my car in tears and promised myself I would never return. I couldn't understand why they felt I was a threat to other people's health. Let's face it: someone who wears bare feet doesn't cough into their foot or pick their nose with their toes and then shake someone's hand with their feet. They don't touch railings, door handles, toilet seats, sinks or countertops and then eat their lunch with their feet when they haven't been washed, like a lot of people I've seen do with their hands. It was ridiculous to think we lived in Canada and our society judged people based on what they wore on their feet.

Take a moment and ask yourself these questions: What makes being barefoot unhygienic? Why is it so disgusting? What is insulting about it? What does it have to do with eating with your hands in a restaurant?

How to Wear Bare Feet

Think about your answers and about how you are judging yourself and others. Are you being realistic about what you believe to be socially unacceptable—not just with being barefoot, but anything in life?

Our society has been duped into believing myths about laws and health code regulations. For example, did you know it's not illegal to drive barefoot? I heard a story about how that urban legend evolved. It all started back in the 1960s with truck drivers who used their CB radios to communicate with each other. If they got stopped by a police officer for a small driving or safety infraction, they would get on their CB radio and, using their lingo, tell another driver. They would say, "Hey, I got caught driving barefoot." It had nothing to do with what they had on their feet. Since many other people at the time had CBs, they heard the truckers, and they interpreted it to mean it was illegal to drive barefoot. People think there's a law, although they've never been told this officially. Take note: it is not illegal to drive barefoot in Canada or the USA.[2]

On top of that, it's proven to be more dangerous to drive with shoes on, especially high heels, flip-flops, heavy boots and platform shoes. You can't possibly feel the pedals. As we age, reaction times slow down, but if you've been exposing your bare soles to the ground, you can be sure your reaction time is much faster. Why not give it a try!

The resistance to allowing my bare feet in stores and restaurants gave me an idea. Could I design a shoe without a sole?

Note: If you are asked to leave a restaurant or store, there is an organization in the USA called Barefoot Living Society. It has a library of letters and can research the laws in various states and in Canada.

---

[2] Source: http://www.barefooters.org/driving-barefoot/

Chapter 9

Barefoot Shoes

Whenever I went barefooting in public, I found people to be very curious. Some approached me, wondering where my shoes were: others thought I was flakey. In general people responded to the look of a bare foot far differently (viscerally) than to open sandals or flip flops, which create virtually no additional physical protection or visual barrier. The only difference in their wearing shoes is that their soles are covered and there are straps holding the shoes onto their feet.

One year I got very sick after Christmas; I'd come down with pneumonia. Bedridden and alone, I had no real energy to do anything. It gave me a lot of time to think about what I had experienced when I was barefoot in stores and restaurants. An idea for a soleless shoe had been brewing in my creative mind. I remembered an old teal leather coat I had stored away to donate to a secondhand store; I took it out to look at it. It was perfect for designing a prototype. I cut a piece of the repurposed leather big enough to cover the top of my foot and began cutting around it.

Once I had the basic design, I made straps to go under the arch to hold it on. Then I cut three holes for the toes: one for the big toe, one for the three middle toes and one for the baby toe. I made straps that wrapped around the back of the heel and tied in the front. The very first pair I cut seemed to work perfectly as soleless shoes.

It was important to me that the style adapt to many different types of feet so they were easy to fit. Barefooting always made me feel like dancing and brought out my inner child. Because of this I made leather straps that wrapped around the ankle, like a ballet shoe. They were elegant, feminine and a little sexy, too.

After wear-testing the first pair, I made another and another, until I had the design elements worked out. Then I asked my family and friends to try them and give me some feedback. My friends helped me make them by hand. I named my endeavour Barebottom Shoes and started selling them online for a reduced price, asking people to provide feedback. That helped finance further development.

After a week I was bored with being in bed so much. While I cut out more Barebottom Shoes, I started watching TV. One night an ad mentioned auditions for the hit show *Dragons' Den*, where people present their business ideas to a panel of investors. There was no interest on my part to partake in a reality TV show but, at the same time, I could feel a strong, energetic push on my back encouraging me to go east. I tried to ignore it, but for the next few days I was constantly nudged by the ads on TV and the gentle push on my back. Finally I decided I wanted to get out of the house and visit my grandchildren in Peterborough, Ontario, where, coincidentally, one of the auditions were.

When I got to the *Dragons' Den* auditions in my Barebottom Shoes, two newspapers approached me right away to cover my story, along with a TV station and a radio station. I pitched to a couple of producers and passed the audition. They scheduled the actual pitch in front of the Dragons a few months later. Around five thousand businesses across Canada apply, 275 people pitch, and around eighty get on the show. I passed the pitch, and they scheduled my segment to be shown on TV. I made it to the *Dragons' Den*, though I didn't get a deal. Everyone on the panel loved the idea but felt it was too early in the product cycle and they didn't want the risk.

So I went to trade shows, yoga festivals and outdoor events to promote the barefoot movement and sell my footwear. Over the first few years I saw thousands of feet. It surprised me how many people were truly embarrassed to take off their socks and shoes to expose their feet. Many people actually apologized for the way their feet looked, and this wasn't only the Canadians! A large percentage of women's toes were mangled and crossed over each other in a triangle shape that could easily squeeze into a sharply pointed shoe. The women complained that their shoes were painful to wear; they were looking for other options.

It was a complete shock to discover how many people had bunions, which make feet look deformed as well. Lots of people had calluses from their shoes, and a huge percentage of women, men, teens and children had fallen arches. Some people could no longer lift their toes up off the ground—they were too stiff—and even more couldn't balance properly at first when they stood in their bare feet. Many told me their feet were often numb (this was possibly due to shoe-induced neuropathy). The general consensus was that people were at a loss about what to do to improve their situation.

The feet are the foundation for the entire body, and most of what I saw was mushy and weak. I felt a deep sense of compassion and responsibility to do something to help people help themselves by redefining footwear. My design for a true barefoot shoe was what was needed.

Barebottom Shoes are sold all over the world. It's a starter shoe for people who aren't ready to completely bare their feet in public. The strap around the arch of the foot provides a feeling of support. They come in suede, deerskin or neoprene. They also offer a sense of style, and they look like a shoe (without a sole). Now I can get into stores and restaurants without being hassled.

Chapter 10

Dr. Emily

One of the first barefoot experts I met was a podiatrist and human-movement specialist from New York City who wrote a book that has become one of my favorites, *Barefoot Strong*. Dr. Emily Splichal focuses on an area of anti-aging medicine known as movement longevity by educating and empowering her patients and other professionals about being barefoot-strong. As she says, "As the only point between the body and the ground, our feet play a critical role in the way in which our body controls and reacts to every upright movement."

She is an internationally renowned educator specializing in barefoot training whom I follow religiously on social media. What she offers freely to her readers is exceptional material: a variety of online courses along with educational videos on fascial fitness and neuromuscular conditioning. In awe of how much stronger my feet became the more I went barefoot, I was inspired by her work. I signed up for her course called Barefoot Training Specialist in Barrie, Ontario, and learned more about the integrated function of the foot.

As much as I learned about barefoot science, I deferred to experience as my primary teacher and continued to experiment with the ground below my feet in the forest. I was now running along logs and hopping across puddles of water in the forest. When I got home from a walk or run in the forest, I had loads of energy, my mind was clear, and I almost always had a smile on my face. I was getting stronger not only physically, but emotionally and mentally as well. It felt like my brain was getting a workout, too.

Since I had learned about the effect of the interoceptors from the Barefoot Professor, I was intrigued to learn more about how our body is designed to look after itself. As Dr. Emily explains,

> Considered one of the most proprioceptive-rich areas of the man body, the plantar foot responds to and can actually anticipate every closed chain movement we do.
>
> In the foot we have two sizes of nerves—small and large—with the smaller nerves being found in the bottom of the foot. Because of the smaller diameter these plantar nerves are able to send signals faster to the Central Nervous System, creating faster response times.

When we cover these nerves, it causes a delay in the time it takes to respond and increases reliance on large nerves in the ankle and lower leg. Our nervous system was designed to be efficient and, according to Dr. Emily, this is one of the key components to movement longevity. She describes walking as a series of falls. When the foot hits the ground, the body is designed to use the impact force as energy for the next step. I always thought I was using muscles to lift up my leg and take a step. In other words, our body has to first perceive the impact and then respond. Who would have thought? According to her, eighty percent of our plantar receptors are sensitive to vibrations and they have the only contact with the ground. They pass that vibration to the muscles, which contract. Shoes, socks, cushioning and extra support weakens our muscles and puts us at risk. She says that if we at least warm up barefoot before a workout, we can decrease injury. I'd strongly recommend you read her book to get more insight.

When I first started walking barefoot, I felt clumsy and awkward. I didn't know whether to put my heel down or my entire foot. Dr. Emily teaches us to walk consciously. Think about how hard your heel lands on the ground and find the rhythm in each step. We should feel the foot strike starting from the outside of the heel then roll to the center of the foot and then off the toes.

> "The fluidity of the motion begins with a subtle heel stroke that should mimic walking on ice or almost flatfooted. Interesting the less dorsiflexion you have in the ankle upon heel strike, the lower the impact forces you will encounter."

You can watch videos on how to assess your own gait, if you have someone film you, at www.youtube.com/ebfafitness.

> "Another great tip I like to give my tendonitis patients is to dorsiflex the great toe upon heel strike. The dorsiflexion of the great toe increases the stiffness of the foot, allowing better transfer of vibrations. This is one of the reasons why impact injury rate is so high in flip-flops or thongs."

Dr. Emily refers to the way our feet gather impact forces. She is seeing impact-related injuries not just in athletes but in people who are getting injured walking to work, or maybe even pilgrims walking the Camino. Our nervous system anticipates impact forces; when there's a mismatch it leads to injury. Concrete tile or marble doesn't transfer efficiently, and the impact transfers through the body. Instead of staying in the soft tissue, it transfers into the bones and causes injuries. To reduce injuries, Dr. Emily suggests we wear shoes that have a zero drop and a lack of support. When I first wore minimalist shoes, I found them to be very comfortable and easy to wear, but it took me a long time to transition to them.

If we have to wear shoes, we can keep the feet strong and flexible and engage foot-to-core integration. She teaches how to do this with "Short Foot" and many other effective exercises at www.barefootstrong.com.

When it comes to orthotics, Dr. Emily says many people benefit from them, but in fact our foot was designed to work on its own.

"Some of the most common conditions treated with orthotics include flat feet, Achilles tendonitis and bunions. But what's amazing is that these are also the most common conditions that benefit the greatest from barefoot training!"

It's a personal decision to go barefoot, at least some of the time. I have had so many profound physical changes since I strengthened the foundation of my entire body that I cannot go back to wearing shoes all the time. There are a few instances, like when I want to dress up and slip into a pair of heels. The problem I have when I wear shoes is that I can't last very long in them and end up taking them off.

Little changes every day have a huge impact on longevity and quality of life. Do you want to be walking in the forest when you are eighty or ninety or one hundred? I do.

Chapter 11

Sole Skin and Sweat

It's easy to wear bare feet. All you do is take off your shoes and socks and you are doing it!

After a couple of years, you too may discover that the skin on the soles of your feet becomes different from the skin on any other part of your body. But rather than growing thicker calluses and blisters—something we might expect from walking around on different terrain barefoot—the opposite happens: your feet begin to exfoliate. The fact is, we get calluses from our feet rubbing inside shoes or boots.

Wearing shoes and socks keeps our feet warm, often too warm, and this sets up a perfect breeding ground for bacteria. For most of my adult life I've had dry, cracking skin on the soles of my feet. When I started walking barefoot, particularly on wet grass, the skin on my feet became very soft, like the palm of my hand. You'd be forgiven for thinking soft skin is an invitation for blisters to form—which is exactly what happened on the Camino when my socks got wet and I had to keep walking to finish my day—but it doesn't happen that way when barefooting.

Walking on the grass, in the forest, through mud and over rocks and roots that were often slippery, the skin on your feet seems to adapt quickly. The skin seems to accept its new role, and grip is better than with shoes. When I wore hiking boots in the forest, I would avoid stepping on slippery rocks or roots and instead land on the dirt, where I had more grip. In bare feet I like to jump from rock to rock, trusting the skin on my soles will adapt to the environment. There's less danger of slipping or falling; it's like having an incredible superhero-like grip.

Last winter I lived in Toronto for five months. During that time I was mostly barefoot and there wasn't a lot of snow. When I walked on concrete or pavement, the skin on my feet immediately changed, becoming rough and callused. I didn't like the way the soles of my feet looked when I was on a man-made surface, but whenever I was on the belly of Mother Earth, the skin was quite soft and beautiful. I was fascinated by this, so I would often test my skin's abilities by quickly changing terrains and then feeling the difference or even observing the skin. According to my calculations, this sole skin was adapting in milliseconds, and it responded one hundred percent of the time.

Howell, the Barefoot Professor, explains the unique features of what he calls "foot-skin" almost exactly the way I was experiencing it. He says our feet have immutable prints to improve grip and increase traction for walking and running.

> Like the tread on a car tire, those skin folds augment friction to better enable us to grasp the ground and reduce slipping. Unlike car tires which go 'bald' and must be replaced, our skin is self-replenishing, prints and all. Of course, our skin prints are rather useless inside a shoe and many shoe soles are smooth and extremely slippery by comparison, especially under wet conditions.

How to Wear Bare Feet

I can attest to this, as I feel the gripping function when I'm running on rocks in the forest.

One fall day when I was walking in the forest barefoot, the soles of my feet turned a deep orange color that I couldn't scrub off. I posted a question on one of the barefoot pages I followed, asking if anyone knew why this was happening. One man from Germany told me to think of the word for "Christmas tree"—Tannenbaum.

In the autumn, oak leaves are the last to fall to the ground, and they are always orange. It's because they have tannins in them. These are the same tannins that are used to tan the hides of animals for leather, and by walking on the leaves I was naturally tanning the soles of my feet in preparation for the coming winter.

At the same time all the animals in the forest with paws were also preparing for the winter ahead. Is it possible that Mother Earth has considered the needs of both humans' bare feet and the paws of animals in the natural cycle of the trees in the forest? I'd like to think so. Based on this, I could trust that my feet would take care of me wherever I was in the world.

Our hands, head and feet are the sweatiest parts of our body. According to Howell,[3] the function of the skin on the feet is to produce microdroplets of sweat to evaporate and remove heat from the body. When we wear socks and shoes, the sweat becomes trapped and breeds bacteria and fungi. Often this results in athlete's foot, for which the best treatment is to go barefoot. I've suspected this, but he confirmed that being in shoes all the time leads to difficulty in regulating body temperature, a condition he calls hot-foot syndrome.

---

[3] See Appendix. http://barefootprof.blogspot.ca/2010/11/special-skin-on-your-feet.html

Chapter 12

Earthing

Some time ago I bought a book called *Earthing*. The authors' research showed that the earth maintains a negative electrical charge on its surface. Our bodies are bioelectrical, and when we are in direct contact we can conduct electricity; it brings us to the same electrical potential as the earth. Since most people wear shoes with plastic or rubber soles, they are cut off from this source of energy.

"Earthing is a fast-growing movement based upon the discovery that connecting to the Earth's natural energy is foundational for vibrant health."[4]

In the book, the authors explain how it works. A charge can be conducted through leather but not through the man-made materials that typically comprise soles on shoes. They claim that earthing positively affects heart rate, inflammation, sleep and the autonomic nervous system and reduces the effects of stress. It also reduces the effect of EMFs (electromagnetic frequencies).

We have positively charged molecules in our body that should be neutralized by negative charges to stop them from damaging our healthy cells. We get some of these antioxidants in food, but it's not enough to stabilize our immune system.

---

[4] www.earthing.com

Negative charges are always available through the earth and are delivered from your feet to different parts of your body. The book claims that, because of this, if you are grounded you are less stressed. Earthing helps to reduce inflammation, which is the base of all disease. I was fascinated by this, relating to their ideas from my own experience. When connected to the earth, I had often felt a surge of energy through my body—even before I read the book. I feel healthier now, and the chronic eczema I had on my legs healed.

One of the authors of *Earthing* confirms the positive effects of grounding. Dr Jospeh Mercola says, "This simple process of grounding is one of the most potent antioxidants we know of. Grounding has been shown to relieve pain, reduce inflammation, improve sleep, enhance well being, and much, much more. Unfortunately, many living in developed countries are rarely grounded anymore."[5]

The more you are barefoot in the forest, the more visceral the experience is. I often felt an immense sense of imp-like freedom. Other times, it was work. Awareness of the sensory feedback of the sensations under my feet expanded the experience of the temperature, textures, the states of the ground, mud, dampness, humidity, vegetation and more.

Yet, my biggest fear, even to this day, is stepping in dog poop.

---

[5] http://articles.mercola.com/sites/articles/archive/2015/11/21/grounding-effects.aspx

Chapter 13

Ecotherapy and Hydrotherapy

More and more people, professionals among them, have reawakened to the benefits of ecotherapy, going outside and spending time in nature, as a component of integrative medicine, which looks at our health as a whole. It includes the physical, mental, emotional and spiritual realms. It's a nature-based method of physical and psychological healing treatments where the inseparable human-nature relationship matters. It includes latest scientific understandings of our universe together with indigenous wisdom of our ancestors.

> At his office in Washington, D.C., Robert Zarr, a pediatrician, writes prescriptions for parks. He pulls out a prescription pad and scribbles instructions—which park his obese or diabetic or anxious or depressed patient should visit, on which days, and for how long—just as though he were prescribing medication.[6]

When we don't get enough time outdoors we get "nature deficit disorder." Dr. Zarr is on the edge of a leading group of health-care professionals who are medicalizing nature and using local parks to

---

[6] https://www.theatlantic.com/magazine/archive/2015/10/the-nature-cure/403210/

prescribe healing. Today, when an ecotherapy treatment is recommended by a doctor, such as listening to a bird singing or spending twenty minutes in the park without your cell phone, the 'prescription' carries more weight.

The Japanese have been studying the effects of being in the presence of trees since the early 1980s, and it has become an important element of preventive health care and healing in Japanese medicine. "Researchers primarily in Japan and South Korea have established a robust body of scientific literature on the health benefits of spending time under the canopy of a living forest."[7] They call the practice forest bathing, or Shinrin Yoku, and it supports what we've known intuitively: simply being in the forest is medicine. Some of the benefits include boosted immune-system functioning, with an increase in the count of the body's Natural Killer (NK) cells, as well as reduced blood pressure, reduced stress and increased ability to focus, even in children with ADHD.

Hydrotherapy, on the other hand, is a series of health-promoting treatments using water. Living on the lake afforded me frequent opportunities to be in the water, immersed in the benefits of aquatic treatments. I especially liked to go for a swim or walk in the cold water after my walks in the forest. As winter approached I would step into the cold water of the lake and walk around the shallow section, lifting each foot out completely out of the water before stepping down. A friend informed me there was a name for what I was doing. It's called Kneipping, and is also referred to as water walking. As cold water temporarily narrows the blood vessels and is followed by vascular expansion when the foot comes out of the water, it promotes

---

[7] http://www.shinrin-yoku.org/shinrin-yoku.html

circulation throughout the body. This strengthens immune defenses, stimulates the circulatory and nervous system as well as metabolism and invigorates the body. No wonder I was feeling fantastic.

It was a Bavarian priest, Sebastian Kneipp (1821–1897), who rediscovered the healing power of water that the ancient Romans used. He created a hydrotherapy treatment that uses immersion baths and therapy experiences that apply hot and cold water to the skin to stimulate blood flow. Today it is offered in wellness centers and spas all over the world, particularly in Europe, because of its natural healing effects on the metabolic system and the immune system. Fortunately for me, I was in an environment that offered hydrotherapy in a natural state. Several other applications of hydrotherapy, with benefits and health warnings, can be found at the website *www.kneipp.com*.[8]

An easy way to integrate barefoot hydrotherapy into your daily practice is to try Kneipping but not everyone has a river or a lake they can access. Be creative. You can do it in the bathtub too!

The art of dew walking is one of the easiest ways to access the healing powers of the earth. All you do is walk barefoot in the morning on dew-covered grass. It feels refreshing, and by stepping in wet grass you also get the benefits of earthing, discharging the static electricity from EMFs that we gather. It sounded pretty easy and made sense, so I started right away. It was important for me to create a ritual or practice, so I decided to do it each morning as soon as I woke up. The first time it was a cool fall day; I lasted just a few minutes, since the grass was extremely cold. At first it was liberating and sent a light buzz through my body. Since I wasn't accustomed to having

---

[8] https://www.kneipp.com/us_en/natures-expert/water-cure/walking-barefoot-and-dew-walking/

cold feet, I would usually put extra socks on under my waterproof winter boots to keep my feet dry and warm. It was a sensation I slowly got used to. It was the first time in many years, maybe in my life, that I paid attention to the sensation of wet coldness on my feet as a pleasant experience, and in time I grew to love the practice of dew walking.

Lastly, there is a growing movement that focuses on climate change. Ecosexual is all about being one with the earth and treating it as your mother. Performance artists Annie Sprinkle and her partner, Beth Stephens, are the co-creators who are trying to make the environmental movement more fun.

This was just the beginning of my cold-water-therapy journey. I seriously questioned how I could barefoot throughout the year in Canada, considering our cold winters.

Chapter 14

Snow Bathing

Winter was upon us, and I could no longer put my bare feet directly on the ground, which I found to be very discouraging. The cottage floor was always cold. At first I was wearing socks to keep my feet warm, an old habit I couldn't seem to break, even with all I had learned about the exteroceptors on the soles of my feet. There were trees all around me and the lake in front of me, yet I would look outside with a longing to be barefoot in the forest. The best I could do was get my snowshoes on and head to my favorite forest for some Shinrin Yoku. At least being in the presence of trees made me feel at peace. Still, I felt disconnected from the earth now that she was covered in snow.

Often a strong northeasterly wind off the lake added to the chill, and the temperature could dip to minus 4 to minus 22 Fahrenheit in January or February. It seemed absurd to consider going barefoot in the snow, even at the beginning of the winter, so I resigned myself to wearing boots when I went outside.

One day, I stood at the back door. I was greatly tempted to step outside in my bare feet. I was close to setting my foot down on the cold snow, but I abruptly stopped myself, convinced that going out there barefoot would be reckless. Everything I had learned and read to that point said that footwear was meant for extreme conditions, so I went back and put my socks and boots on, surmising that it was too dangerous. I could get frostbite.

When I got to town, I met a friend who saw I was wearing boots. He teased me, saying, "Too bad you can't go barefoot in the snow. I guess you'll have to wait for spring." I'd fallen into the same kind of fear-induced thinking as most people, even though I knew how the sensory receptors worked in harmony with the brain to protect me. This, along with the thought of waiting four more months before I could touch the earth, was enough to motivate me to decide to literally step outside of my comfort zone.

Once home I took my boots and socks off in the car and ran barefoot into the cottage as fast as I could, laughing delightedly all the way. It was so liberating to feel the cold on my feet that I dropped my boots at the back door and went outside again. This time I moved my feet around in the ankle-deep snow, feeling the cool lightness of the snowflakes on the top of my foot. I laughed again, and I felt like a child. After about thirty seconds I went indoors and warmed my feet up. That was the beginning of what I now affectionately call "snow bathing."

Eventually I stopped wearing socks or slippers around the house, mostly because it was too much work. Yes, my feet got very cold at first, but I tried to think of the sensory feedback to my brain. Then one day I noticed I wasn't feeling cold. The skin on the bottom of my feet was cool, not cold. The top of my feet was actually warm to the touch.

It was still early in the winter, and there were patches of exposed dirt on the ground where the snow had melted. Each day I went outside and put my soles on the earth as many times as I could. You can imagine my joy as I discovered something new that was happening

How to Wear Bare Feet

in my barefoot world. I became more respectful and trusting that my feet would take care of me, whether the situation was extreme or not. I didn't have to manage keeping my feet warm, but I had to be smart about it. There was an element of danger walking in the snow.

During all of my athletic life, until I started rowing, I think I was always fighting with my body to make it do something I wanted it to do. No pain, no gain. Once I learned the technical movement of rowing, I thought I would train harder and row faster. My coach would often say, "The problem with rowers is that they slow the boat down." In other words, we get in the way of its design, which is to move quickly, because we think we can control it. I discovered it was possible to surrender to the crew and to the boat; then it moved extremely fluidly and fast. Once our crew of eight rowers aligned with the boat and rowed technically well, we were able to win the FISA World Masters Rowing Regatta.

Barefooting follows a similar philosophy. One must practice walking on different natural terrains to wake up the neural pathways to the brain, and then absolutely surrender to them to do their job.

The approach I took was to expose my feet to the cold or snow for a few minutes every day and gradually extend the exposure. The sensory nerve receptors became very efficient at communicating to the central nervous system that it was extremely cold outside and my feet were in danger of getting frostbite. The major organs were checked to ensure they were all warm and out of danger, and the command was sent from the central nervous system to thin the blood so it would rush to my feet and extremities to warm them up quickly. How amazing is that?

Today when I go outside in the snow, initially my feet don't feel the cold at all. It takes about ten minutes at 14 Fahrenheit for me to notice how cold it is. The longer I stay out in the cold, the easier it is for my body to adapt to extreme temperatures. My brain is a depository of input. Once it has experienced a sensation, it knows how to adapt better the next time.

I learned about Wim Hof, who is known as the Ice Man because of his Guinness World Record for being immersed in freezing cold water for over two hours. He teaches people how to raise consciousness and improve health. The Wim Hof Method combines specific breathing techniques, cold exposure and specific physical exercises. It's a natural method to improve health and well being. The cold-shower training is the first practice he recommends in his ten-week program, and I've done it. You take a cold shower each day for thirty seconds, practice breathing and do some basic exercises. Try not to stress or react and let your body and feet adapt to the environment. I noticed changes right away. Visit his website to take a free mini-class: www.wimhofmethod.com

During that first winter there were several changes in my body. The fat pad on the soles of my feet got thicker over time. If I stood on a cold surface for any length of time, the pad would swell, seemingly in an effort to keep my feet away from the cold and protect them. Then my feet would heat up for the next few hours, keeping me extra warm. It seems that my hands responded to the cold weather training as well, because I no longer need winter mitts all the time.

There is another kind of fat in your body that keeps you warm. I read an online article about some marathoners who were training in the cold to increase the amount of brown fat in their body. Ever since I started snow bathing I've noticed that I loose about five pounds at the beginning of the winter and maintain my desired weight throughout the season.

Spending time in the cold makes your brown fat more active, and could even cause you to grow new brown-fat cells, according to a 2014 study conducted by National Institutes of Health researchers and published in the journal *Diabetes*. Unlike regular old white fat, which stores calories, mitochondria-packed brown-fat cells burn energy and produce heat. It was once thought that, in humans, only babies had brown fat. But in 2009, researchers found small amounts of brown fat in adults. What's more, they found that people with lower body mass indexes (BMIs) tended to have more brown fat. This finding suggests "a potential role of brown [fat] in adult human metabolism," the researchers wrote in their findings.[9]

Imagine that. The foundation of a healthy, fulfilling life could be in the soles of our feet.

---

[9] https://www.livescience.com/49652-what-is-brown-fat-facts.html

Chapter 15

Anti-Aging and Movement Longevity

There are no real negative side effects to barefooting. It reverses the aging process, improves brain function, boosts self-esteem and makes you feel happy. It's natural medicine. I'm reminded of a quote I often use in my workshops or life-coaching program. It's from the Buddha. "There is no way to happiness. Happiness is the way." The soles of my feet and all the sensory receptors help me to 'feel' my happiness. Together we walk, sole to soul into the forest of love. There isn't one single scientific measurement that can accurately tell me when I'm happy with life, with my weight, with the way I am aging, with the way my brain is working, if my heart is open, or any measurement of my happiness. The truth is within us.

After I ditched my shoes, my bare feet were resting completely flat on the ground and my Achilles tendon had to extend more so that my heel could touch the ground. By dropping my heels to zero, I was forced to tilt backward ever so slightly and engage my core muscles. This allowed my chin to settle into position more naturally and forced me to relax my shoulders for better alignment. As time passed, my back got stronger and my posture improved. I could sit up without back support for long periods of time without any discomfort. I was getting the benefits of doing a workout without having to go to the gym, and I was outside.

When we have good posture, our entire body is physically aligned and our organs, muscles, tendons, ligaments, bones, spine and other components can work more efficiently. Our body can work more efficiently on important matters like regulating blood flow or avoiding injury or falls. The benefits I was receiving from barefooting were starting to look more like an approach to longevity and anti-aging than feeling closer to nature.

So what changed for me physically, after a few years of a barefoot lifestyle? I was no longer stiff when I got up in the morning, and my arthritis was virtually gone. The temperature of my body regulated itself, and I wasn't cold all the time. The arches in my feet actually went back to the height and spring they had in my early twenties. The skin on the soles of my feet could adjust to the environment within seconds. My bunion wasn't as pronounced. I got rid of the athlete's foot, and my feet didn't smell anymore. I found out you get calluses from shoes, not from the ground. My bite improved, and I hardly ever grind my teeth. My posture improved, and my neck wasn't sore anymore. The vaginal atrophy I experienced reversed. My allergies to dogs and cats ceased, and I rarely had any asthma at all. My knees touched each other when I stood up, a sign of perfect alignment.

There have been a few surprises, too. My double chin has gone away. My balance has drastically improved, and I'm no longer afraid of heights. My brain is functioning at a higher level and I remember more than I used to. I am at my perfect natural weight. I am more flexible than I've been in thirty years, and I can almost do the splits again. I look younger. I have more energy. My hair is thicker. I can digest foods more easily. I am physically stronger. My ankles are thinner and I have more defined muscle in my calves. The inflammation in my body has gone down, especially in my face, hands, wrists, legs and belly. My craving for sweets has diminished. I'm more sensual. I can stand on the balls of my feet for long periods of time. I've been doing yoga on and off for twenty-seven years, but now I can hold postures longer than ever without falling over. Of course none of these are scientifically proven, but I can attest to them.

Instead of constantly asking my body if I need more water, less fruit, more vegetables, less juice, more greens, less sleep, more exercise, and so on, I am guided about the nutrients my body needs and how much to eat, how much sleep I need, when to go back to nature, and when I'm not healthy.

My body absorbs nutrients from the earth and I intuitively eat or drink whatever else is required in small quantities. In the past I would often eat too much because I honestly had no idea what my body needed to sustain itself. As a seasoned barefooter, I know when to stop eating. It's not something I have to grapple with consciously; I just stop eating. The Buddha says, "Enough is too much." I've finally learned what enough is, and I'm loving it.

Katy Bowman talks about the high percentage of seniors who are afraid of falling. They believe as they get older they are getting weaker rather than stronger. It's common practice to remove things that can become obstacles from their living space so there is less risk of falling, which actually puts them at more risk. If they change the way they move, with fear their gait shortens, and that affects their movement.

Chapter 16

Nutritional Mud

My absolute favorite ground to walk or run barefoot on is the mud. Some would pay dearly for a Swedish or Moorish mud bath at a spa, but I prefer to connect with Mother Earth directly by putting my feet in the natural mud found in forests, jungles, parks and even my backyard. Mud is nourishing for our entire body and has an abundance of mineral content, nutrients, beneficial micro-organisms, iron, magnesium, calcium, manganese and more.

I have found that the soles of my feet absorb enough moisture from the mud to quench my thirst, so I don't have to carry as much water. When I'm in the forest on a warm day, I look for mud to step into, as it also cools down my body.

Craig Chalquist, the chair of the East-West Psychology Department at the California Institute of Integral Studies, says, "If you hold moist soil for twenty minutes… the soil bacteria begin elevating your mood. You have all the antidepressant you need in the ground."[10]

Mud also reminds me of my childhood. I grew up in the inner city in Toronto. In our neighborhood, the lawns weren't manicured and our backyard had a lot of dirt instead of grass. I had six siblings.

---

[10] https://www.theatlantic.com/magazine/archive/2015/10/the-nature-cure/403210/

My mother let us go barefoot whenever we wanted to. I remember that everyone in the family used to tease me about being so clumsy. Mum would often say that I could trip over a toothpick. I didn't understand how I could do cartwheels on a balance beam and at the same time trip and fall down on my way to school. Today I understand that I was likely clumsy because I was wearing shoes and couldn't feel the ground below my feet.

Mum would often bring out a jug of water, a bowl and spoons and encourage my sister, Pattie, and I to make mud pies. We would spend hours making them. One time she gave us some chocolate chips to put on the top of our creations. The mud pies that day were dark and extra moist, so they stuck together. We were so proud of them we decided to invite our little sisters, Donna, Lorie, Joanne and baby Kelly, to a tea party with an imaginary teapot and cups. Even our two-year-old brother, Larry, joined in.

Mum saw what we were doing and gave us a blanket to lay on the dirt/grass. Pattie was good at organizing, so she got all the little kids sitting in a perfect circle with the tray of decorated mud pies in the center. We both went around the circle and poured imaginary tea. Pattie announced that no one was to eat a mud pie until everyone got one. We carefully doled them out, and each child gently held them in their palms. Our siblings were all under the age of eight, and they all patiently waited until everyone was served.

The party started, and all the mud pies went into the kids' mouths. To our surprise they actually took a bite. You can imagine their reaction when they tasted the dirt. They made disgusted faces and started trying to spit out the mud stuck to their tongue and the inside of their mouth. The littlest ones began crying, and the older kids helped scoop the mud out with their fingers. Pattie and I jumped up to help. We carried kids into the house, and Mum grabbed a chair and moved it to the sink. She washed out their mouths with water from the tap.

Pattie and I thought we'd be in big trouble for giving the little kids dirt. When we finished cleaning everyone's mouths and the tears dried up, Mum looked at the two of us with a grin. All she said was, "It's okay, girls. You have to eat a peck of dirt before you die." We all started to laugh.

I'm forever grateful to my mother, who is now eighty-five years old, because she was never afraid to let us play in nature, eat mud, go barefoot, find insects, bring animals home, climb trees and explore our natural surroundings without fear. She was an inspiration as I raised my own children with the same values. Today I am living proof that her teachings were important.

Wherever I am in the world, I taste the mud in the forest. The most delicious so far is in the cloud forest in Mindo, Ecuador. Apparently the first few inches of black earth there is the most nutrient-dense in the world. The next best to that is Muskoka mud!

Chapter 17

Barefoot Babies

Watching my grandkids in their bare feet is a truly wonderful experience for me. Seeing them run along rocks and jump and play by the water at the cottage reminds me that every minute they are out of shoes is one more minute they are developing their feet to be strong and flexible later in life. This summer I watched my three-and-a-half-year-old grandson climb a tree. He went up about eight feet without a care in the world. His parents have always let their kids play barefoot and encourage them not to be afraid. His dad took him to a rock-climbing gym and, after they put the harness on him, he climbed up the entire wall without stopping. He had the attention of every adult climber in the gym.

The beauty of seeing that is knowing the parents or grandparents don't have to rely as much on a young child realizing a dangerous situation: their feet and brain will take care of them and help them recover from any situation faster than the child can think. That means environments are less dangerous, which brings relief to and reduces stress for the parents.

Dr. Phil Maffetone, clinician, coach and innovator who has worked with some of the greatest athletes in the world, talks about the effect of shoes on kids in this article excerpt:

Among the untold problems that wearing shoes can impose in the developing child is the impact on the brain. From a baby's very first delicate steps, each walking and running gait pattern significantly influences brain development. These actions affect lifelong patterns in the nervous system, even beyond the gait and balance mechanisms—they include postural habits, the ability to compensate to physical stresses, and the growth of muscles, bones, ligaments, tendons and other tissues. Normally, with each muscle contraction and relaxation, and every joint movement, important neurological patterns are created by the brain, just like with any memory. Shoes distort this process, and instead, the brain learns and designs irregular patterns of movement throughout the body.[11]

When kids have their bare soles free, they have fun. They exude confidence, balance, agility, stability, playfulness and flexibility in their stride. You can almost determine by their movements how quickly their brain is being sent feedback from the exteroceptors on the soles of their feet. And if a child has a strong foundation, then the rest of the body works efficiently and quickly. These nerve endings are developed at infancy and have to last a lifetime.

Some people would call me a senior because I am over sixty, but I am no longer afraid of falling, something that haunted me for ten years after I had one bad fall. I was afraid because my reaction time was so slow I couldn't depend on it. If I tripped on something and started to fall, by the time I realized I was off balance it was too late.

---

[11] https://philmaffetone.com/kids-shoes/

How to Wear Bare Feet

The fall was in play, and all I could do was try to minimize the injury. Since I've been barefooting on uneven surfaces, mostly in the forest, I've experienced potential falls. Instead of me noticing belatedly that I was off balance, my brain would already be working on rebalancing my body thanks to messages my exteroceptors had sent.

One time a friend was with me when I experienced my recovery. I tripped going over a log on the forest floor and, when I started to fall, my right arm straightened and suddenly swung up over my head. I was upright, and then I did a 180-degree turn on one foot, paused for a second, then did another 180-degree turn. My arm came down (on its own) and I took a step forward on the path as though nothing had happened at all. That experience solidified complete respect for and confidence in my feet. I'm convinced they will take care of me and keep me out of harm. That is their job. When we wear shoes, we get in the way of the natural sensory-feedback process, making falls more likely for toddlers, children and adults.

Many current studies conclude that shoes are the culprit behind loss of foot mobility and natural gait. Children's feet become weak, and they lose normal foot structure and function by the time they are seven or eight years old, according to podiatrist Dr. William A. Rossi.

"In any shoe-wearing society, by age eight or nine, the toes of most children have lost up to 50 percent of their natural prehensile and functional capacity. They are no longer strong, finger-like, ground grasping organs but weak [appendages] at the end of the foot," he says.

If you were to think about how we walk and how limiting it is to be in shoes with thick, inflexible soles with no room for movement in the toes, the arches or the heels, you would avoid 'normal' footwear. Shoes hold the entire foot in one position. Because the shoe has traction, the foot has to stop to break with each step. Why would we expose our children to this if we knew how much it was hurting the function of their feet and, ultimately, their entire body?

In bare feet, most kids will look where they are going and avoid common dangers. We don't want to scare children about the environment but rather encourage them to explore. Depending on where they are, caregivers may need to prescreen the area for safety. Otherwise, you can trust their feet will watch over them.

Chapter 18

Primal Running

It made perfect sense to me that the entire posture of my body was adjusting to the shift in alignment, since my heels had been raised by up to one inch in shoes or boots and up to three inches in heels. My bare feet now rested completely flat on the ground. This minor shift meant that the heels weren't being elevated for eight to ten hours a day, and this was throwing my posture off. By dropping my heels to zero, I was forced to tilt backward ever so slightly and engage my core muscles. This allowed my chin to settle into position more naturally and forced me to drop my shoulders.

Not long after I started walking in the forest, I had a moment that redefined running for me. It was a gorgeous sunny day. I was alone in the shadows of the sunlight coming through the trees. Out of the blue, I was moved to leap over some roots and I landed on the balls of my feet. Then I jumped onto a log, about a foot in diameter, and I moved along it effortlessly, my arms moving out to the side and then above my head. Landing in some mud, I squished my toes into it as I moved forward, leaping onto solid ground.

It wasn't running as I knew it. It felt raw, natural, graceful, and even tribal. I imagined I was a gazelle and quickened my pace, lifting my knees higher and higher. Soon it developed into an improvised dance with my hands tickling the branches I passed, tapping the trunks of the trees and allowing the warm air to tickle my face as it passed by me. I felt completely free.

My improvisational interpretation of the wooded terrain developed into a form of forest parkour where I was moving through each stage in the moment it was presented. I felt alive, connected, fluid, natural and very, very happy that I was trusting my feet to move me through the forest this way. I wasn't afraid of falling, slipping, losing my balance or tripping over something. I was a tribal movement artist in the forest.

Barefoot running is actually gentler and smoother than running in padded shoes. The foot lands lightly in more of a mid-strike, allowing the three arches in your foot to act as springs to deflect the load and shock to the rest of your body. It feels so natural and free.

After I read Chris McDougall's book *Born to Run*, I started thinking I wanted to run an ultra marathon in my bare feet one day. After I read another fascinating post by the Barefoot Professor about the skin on the soles of our feet and how it differs from the rest of our body, I was convinced I could do it. See the paper on page 85 that describes the skin on the soles of our feet and how it is designed to protect us—but only when we are barefoot!

His research made sense to me. Some of it is scientific, but he refers to something I felt I knew. When I turned sixty, I ran my first ultra marathon, barefoot: The Finger Lakes 50s, which is a fifty-kilometer race in the national forest in New York. I would consider this distance only because I was barefoot and I knew my feet were strong enough to carry me over uneven terrain without fear of injury. Feeling the earth beneath my feet was incredibly calming and tribal. I started training by running through forested paths. Being among the trees gave me the sense I was welcomed as a part of the natural world rather than as a guest. Had I been wearing shoes, I know I would have felt disconnected, unsure and concerned about falling. It's possible I would have been in significant pain, worrying about getting blisters or twisting my ankle.

Being barefoot, I had to be extremely alert and focused on getting out of the way of my feet, trusting they would be able to maneuver the rocks and roots. It was a mental challenge to let go of control and of managing each step, to instead be present in the barefoot dance on the forest floor.

Ryan Smith, a barefoot-running coach from Kentucky, read a post of mine about my plan to run an ultra. He contacted me and offered to coach me complimentarily. Of course I was incredibly grateful, and we started to work together right away. He suggested that, since I was running barefoot, I should focus on eating natural foods, not the Gu Energy Gel and electrolyte drinks that other runners tend to use throughout the day. He shared his philosophy with me.

> The biggest challenge I see with so many endurance athletes: they are disconnected from the ground they run on, the food they eat, and sounds that surround them. Instead they run on an artificial surface to protect them from an artificial surface while taking in artificial food-like substances, while listening to artificial sounds to drown out the voices in their head telling them to stop. It just doesn't make sense.

On the day of the race, it was about 68 Fahrenheit. We were in the cool forest, protected from the sun. For the first twenty-five kilometers I consumed only a four-ounce bottle of water with some Himalayan salt in it. I drank a half cup of water at each of the five water stations but didn't overhydrate. I ate dehydrated berries, nuts, hemp seeds, chia seeds, tortilla wraps with sesame butter and raw honey and my favorite food of all, maple syrup. I managed to run most of it and, by the time I reached the end of the first loop, I was pretty tired.

At the beginning of my second twenty-five-kilometer loop, the balls of my feet were tender from all the rock on the forest path and the large gravel stones on the road, so I put on a pair of Barebottoms with a demi-sole of thin leather that covered only the ball of my foot for protection. It didn't occur to me that the soles of my feet would have to adjust to this sensory input, and within a few minutes I tripped over a tree root.

I got up immediately and kept moving, being a little more aware of the environment. I had stubbed my toe and it was throbbing, but I tried not to think of it as pain and instead focused on the sensation as neither good nor bad. Magically, I recovered very quickly, and the sensory nerve receptors adapted to the environment, too. The next day my toe was swollen, purple and possibly broken. I couldn't put shoes on, but I could still walk perfectly fine barefoot.

In the early stages of training, I always took old shoes with me on a run, just in case. Then I increased my barefoot distance slowly, until I got to the distance I had set as my new goal. You absolutely must take your time transitioning to being totally barefoot; otherwise, you will experience injuries.

I finished the race. I was the second-slowest runner that day out of a couple of hundred people. What I didn't know was that they have a prize for the fastest runner in each age category. That day there were no other sixty-to-sixty-nine-year-old women running, so I won first place by default!

Chapter 19

Barefoot on the Camino

Very few pilgrims have walked barefoot on the Camino in recent times. I've been walking this pilgrimage since 2001, both alone and leading groups. Over the last six years, I have been walking it barefoot, mostly guiding ten-day walks. On average we cover twelve miles a day. Some of the Camino path is made of dirt trails through the forest and of gravel tracks, and at times you walk on pavement or concrete. It's best to avoid walking on flat, hard surfaces in bare feet, and instead walk on the side of the road where the terrain is more natural and soft. When I prepare to walk the Camino barefoot, I spend a lot of time in the forest. Because of the rugged winding paths, the exteroceptors on my feet constantly signal my brain to adjust my balance, transfer my weight, absorb any shock, lift my knees, so I don't trip, can avoid sharp objects and move smoothly.

I've been coaching people to walk the Camino for several years. Now that you've read most of this book, you have an in-depth understanding of how debilitating shoes or hiking boots are for long walks.

With everything I have learned and experienced firsthand, my advice to you is to wear shoes with as little support as you can manage. This is especially important while preparing for the Camino. I urge you to migrate into minimalist shoes. Start wearing them at least six months before you embark on the Camino.

Check out Katy Bowman's book *Whole Body Barefoot: Transitioning Well to Minimal Footwear*. She offers exercises that will strengthen your feet and offers a recommendation on how to migrate to minimalist shoes.

Introducing barefoot training into the regular walking program involves a simple adjustment of the time you spend shod. Let's begin with a few simple guidelines. Wear comfortable shoes or walking sandals with a little extra space in the toe box for swelling or a downward thrust. Don't wear boots unless you absolutely need support. Do cross-training such as running, yoga and Pilates, swim and, of course, walk everyday.

Be gentle. Your entire body is adapting to a zero drop after decades of wearing heels and supportive shoes. Some of your muscles have already atrophied, so you'll need to retrain them. If you've been wearing footwear with arch support, then your metatarsals have to learn how to spring again. This takes time and practice.

When I was shifting to a barefoot lifestyle, I did it gradually, over a year. In the beginning I always brought a pair of my old comfy runners, or walking sandals with cushion and support, on my training walks and on the Camino. It gave me the security of having shoes, just in case, but also I'd have something to change into if my feet or body became unbearably sore.

Many pilgrims experience foot, knee and hip injuries on the Camino and come home in worse shape than when they left. The goal is always to walk injury-free while you build strength, flexibility, balance and reinforce the sensory neural pathways to a responsive brain. Twenty-five percent of all the muscles in our body are in our feet. Barefooting is like exercise for the whole body. That said, the most important advice I can give you is to GO SLOW.

How to Wear Bare Feet

It's ideal if you can walk on grass, dirt, stone or the forest floor. Your bare feet always prefer the most natural, uneven environments. If you are in the city, try to walk on the grass beside the sidewalk or in a park. The more natural the terrain is, the more exercise it provides the small muscles in your feet. You'll ultimately become a barefoot-strong pilgrim.

To get started I suggest you go barefoot for five minutes at the beginning of your walk, put your shoes on for twenty to thirty minutes and then walk barefoot again for five minutes at the end of your walk. Each week, add a bit more time barefoot. Depending on how your body responds to walking without support, you could add five minutes a week and, over time, decrease the amount of time in shoes. Again, go slow. Listen to how your body responds and adapt your walking program. Over time the skin on the soles of your feet will be able to adapt to many different terrains. And, hopefully, there will be no blisters to worry about on your feet.

Even after walking the Camino several times barefoot, I still rely on wearing minimalist shoes or moccasins some of the time because the terrain can be extremely rough and I'm walking long distances over many days. Remember, it's not a competition. Journey at your own pace.

Buen Camino!

Note: If you experience any serious pain or discomfort, pause. Take a day or two off barefoot training to give your body space to heal. If it persists, seek professional medical advice.

Guide

How to Wear Bare Feet

Barefooting is a practice that, like meditation, should be done daily.

This guide is a suggestion of practices you can implement to get started. Always use common sense before you attempt anything. The receptors in your feet will not be effective at protecting you right away, and you will have to build up to that by exposing them to various terrains and sensations. Pay attention and go slowly. If you think you should seek medical attention before you try this, then do so. You are the only one who knows what's right for you.

Ironically, we wear footwear for protection from injury, while, in reality, our greatest source of protection is the two hundred thousand sensory feedback receptors on the soles of our feet. They must be exposed in order to function. When we wear shoes or boots, our feet are being held in a state that is separate from the world and gives us a false sense of security. Very few medical professionals reference this phenomenon; instead, they prescribe orthotics, suggest we wear shoes with more support and thicker heels, and encourage us to avoid potentially dangerous situations like walking barefoot. No wonder many people fear they are out of control in life. They are.

Now that you've learned about the power of going shoeless for strength, balance, longevity, being grounded, feeling in control, and better health, are you ready to integrate it into your life? Once you decide that it is important to you, you can commit to doing it. It's that simple. It's not extra work to add to your busy life. Rather, it's living the way you were meant to.

A good idea is to keep a daily journal so you can review your progress. Pay attention to the changes and write them down. It's extremely helpful to be able to read about the changes you experience and to track your progress.

Hydrate and eat nutritious food. Once you've been practicing barefooting you may find that the earth helps to hydrate you and feed you through the minerals in the soil. Be aware of the temperature, especially in extreme heat or cold. Pay attention to how your feet are responding and adapt as required. If it's too hot or too cold, wear your shoes.

The foot and ankle contain twenty-six bones: one quarter of the bones in the human body. There are thirty-three joints and more than one hundred muscles, tendons and ligaments. Each one gets a workout when you are barefoot.

Honor your feet and the earth, as they honour you.

The How-to-Wear-Bare-Feet Guide

Step 1

Go barefoot at home. Duration/frequency: all the time.

Go barefoot at home always. There is no need for socks, slippers, shoes or any footwear inside. Even if your feet are cold, let them be cold to give the sensory receptors a chance to work with the central nervous system, to thin your blood and send it rushing to your feet to warm them up. You might have to wait ten minutes or so to feel the effects.

Try to think of cold feet simply as a sensation. It's not good or bad. It just is. Pay close attention to other temperature changes and various sensations. This is also an exercise in awareness.

Step 2

Dew walking. Duration/frequency: two minutes — daily.

Go outside first thing every morning and walk on the dewy grass in your bare feet. Be aware of any sensation you experience and try not to think of the temperature or the feeling of the grass as a good or bad sensation. It just is. Teach yourself to let go of past judgments, expectations or reactions about temperature.

Start by walking on the grass for two minutes if the weather is agreeable. If it's winter or extremely cold, be aware of the danger of frostbite and hypothermia. Read Step 5.

Step 3
Shinrin Yoku / forest therapy. Duration/frequency: five to ten minutes — daily.
Stand in the forest barefoot. A forest can be a garden, the woods, a jungle, a park, a tree in your backyard. If you can't get outside to spend time with a tree, you could also bring a potted tree or plants into the house. Don't hesitate to touch the trunks of the trees, and hug them, too. If you are ready for a challenge, try climbing a tree.

Note: A fascinating book about trees is *The Hidden Life of Trees* by Peter Wohlleben. In it he talks about how trees fall in love, have families, communicate through their roots and feel pain. He also says that an electrical charge travels through them, though it moves at a rate of half an inch an hour.

Step 4
Earthing. Duration/frequency: twenty to thirty minutes — two to seven times a week.
Walk or stand on a natural surface such as grass, earth, mud or rock barefoot. If you can't walk, sit in a chair and put your bare feet on the ground. Feel the energy below your feet. You will be gathering negatively charged electrons that will offset the free radicals in your body to reduce inflammation.

Step 5
Snow bathe. Duration/frequency: ten seconds — daily.
If you live in an area where it snows or it gets extremely cold, go outside every day and stand in shallow snow for about ten seconds. It will at least make you laugh, and that's healing, too. Depending on

the temperature and the type of the snow, add a few more seconds when you are ready. Try doing some snowga—yoga barefoot in the snow. Be cautious and aware when it gets cold, as frostbite and hypothermia is a risk. Wet snow has a tendency to draw the heat out of your feet, so spend less time in it. Salt is dangerous because it drops the temperature of the snow or ice to minus 5 Fahrenheit; at this state the atoms break up and turn it into water.

Step 6

Kneipping. Duration/frequency: five minutes — spring, summer, autumn.

If you live near a lake or river that is about knee high in depth, walk in the water. With each step you take, lift your foot out of the water and then drop it back in again. Repeat this with the other foot. Your feet and calves are exposed to cold water and then to warmer air, and this contracts and expands the cells.

Step 7

Walk or run barefoot. Duration/frequency: ten to sixty minutes three times a week — year-round.

Go for a walk and try to find different types of terrains. Look for barefoot-friendly environments like parks and trails. If you live in a place where there are four seasons, adapt to the weather for each season. Think of it as uploading information to your brain about a variety of sensations. The more you have experienced, the more easily and quickly your central nervous system can adapt. In the beginning, always bring minimalist shoes with you. Lift your feet up when you walk. You'll work your quads and core muscles and avoid stubbing your toes and possibly tripping.

Sue Regan Kenney

Other Barefoot Tips

- Walk gently on your feet. Place your heel down and roll to the ball of your foot, pushing off with the big toe.
- Walk on natural surfaces like grass, earth, rock and mud.
- Look where you are going. Watch for broken glass or sharp surfaces. Note: you might even be surprised at how little you actually see.
- Lift your feet when you walk. You'll work your quads and core muscles. Shoes give us the ability to be lazy, so we drag our feet across the ground. If you do this barefoot, the chances for injury are increased.
- Be aware of areas where you might stub your toe. Often the toes become weak and stiff from wearing shoes because they are always being held in the same place by the inside of the shoe or boot.
- Your feet might be sensitive; it might feel painful to walk barefoot at first. Practice in the house and on grass or earth as much as you can.
- Walk as naturally as you can. Try not to make it an effort. It will feel odd at first, because you can actually feel the ground.
- Keep your nails cut short so they don't break if they hit something.
- Wash your feet when you have finished your barefoot walk. Keep a special facecloth at the door so you can wipe your feet, and then wash them with soap and water.
- Be aware of the temperature, especially in extreme heat or cold. Pay attention to how your feet are responding and adapt as required. If it's too hot, wear your shoes.
- Walk on the sunny side of the street; there are fewer bacteria.
- Walk in the rain. You want to give your exteroceptors exposure to as many types of environments as possible.
- If anyone asks you where your shoes are, tell them you are wearing your bare feet—nature's shoes!

Epilogue

Last winter I was working on this book in Mindo, Ecuador. I'd been there for two months as a digital nomad, exploring a cultural experience while towing my Mac. The Great Mother Earth always validates the life lessons I'm given with an actual application in my life. In the case of barefooting, I had made a conscious choice to return to my roots, and because of it my health improved, my body became stronger and more flexible with impeccable balance, and my journey to enlightened consciousness was activated. I had the blessed opportunity to access the mystical and healing powers of the forest through the soles of my feet. She answered my deepest yearning for freedom, tribal connection, awareness and unconditional love.

One day in Ecuador I was coming back from the home of a friend, and I was walking downhill on the shoulder of the road in my bare feet. I looked up to the sky as I followed a bird and tried to figure out what kind it was. I lost my balance and started to fall over. I recalled there was a ditch but didn't have time to think about exactly where I would land. Besides, I knew my feet were already sussing out the situation. I started to fall over a second time, into the ditch. My leg suddenly jerked up, moved my foot to the side of the ditch, where it landed on beautiful, soft mud. My foot slid down the side of the embankment and then stopped, as if it were being directed by a force beyond me.

Immediately I righted myself and landed back on the shoulder of the road. Maybe my soles had made my foot land in the mud because I love it so much, but when I looked into the ditch, I was shocked. I had avoided the worst-case scenario for a barefooter —a broken beer bottle was lying there on its side, its jagged, sharp point right beside my foot. If I had landed on that, it would have sliced my foot open. If I had been in shoes, it's possible I would have stepped on it.

Luckily my bare soles—and responsive sensory receptors—had saved me from a potentially dangerous accident. It reminded me that I had developed a special bond with myself and I could trust my brain was programmed to protect me from danger, illness or pain. I acknowledged my gratitude by being barefoot.

It's a choice to heal our physical bodies and follow the path of our spirit. After experiencing such profound results in the functioning of my body, organs and brain, I wanted to share with the world that it was possible to have a relationship with your physical body and spiritual soul through your feet with love, trust and loyalty.

My barefoot journey to consciousness offered me a chance to explore my inner child—who I found hiding in the forest—through the playfulness of exposing my bare feet to nature. Connecting to my inner child's body, mind and spirit left me in a state of absolute joy.

I listened to the message I received to take people to the forest even though it didn't make sense at the time. By trusting it was valuable and important, and then adopting a barefoot lifestyle, even if it wasn't socially acceptable, I received much more from the forest than I ever expected. I respected the interdependent relationship with nature and stepped onto a path to spirituality through nature. Listening to the elements and to my soul while connected to the ground will always guide me back to my authentic self.

How to Wear Bare Feet

And so this book is my gift to you. It's my way of guiding you back to the forest, to reconnect you with the earth, to helping you find self love, to help you heal your body and mind, and to encourage you to embrace the inner child and have some fun.

Come, take my hand and let's walk together. If we walk together, we can let go of the layers of life, whether it's the emotional or physical, and eventually we will be called to take off the layers that we put over the soles of our feet and expose ourselves to the mud, sole to soul.

I thank the Great Mother Earth for trusting me to guide others on this journey.

Bibliography

Barefoot Running, Michael Sandler with Jessica Lee. RunBare Publishing, 2010.

Barefoot Running Step by Step, Barefoot Ken Bob Saxton. Fair Winds Press, 2011.

Barefoot Strong, Dr. Emily Splichal. New York City: Self-published, 2015.

Born to Run, Christopher McDougall. Vintage, 2011.

Dynamic Aging, Katy Bowman, Joan Virginia Allen. Propriometric Press, 2017.

Earthing, Clinton Ober, Stephen T. Sinatra and Martin Zucker. Basic Health Publications, 2010.

The Barefoot Book: 50 Great Reasons to Kick Off Your Shoes, L. Daniel Howell. Hunter House Inc., 2010.

The Brain That Changes Itself, Norman Doidge. Viking Press, 2007.

The Hidden Life of Trees, Peter Wohlleben. Greystone Books, 2016.

Whole Body Barefoot, Katy Bowman. Propriometric Press, 2015.

~

"Foot Anatomy 101–Biofeedback," Daniel Howell. http://barefootprof.blogspot.com/2011/04/foot-anatomy-101-biofeedback.html, accessed April 1, 2011.

"Foot Anatomy 101–Special Skin on Your Feet," Daniel Howell. http://barefootprof.blogspot.ca/2010/11/special-skin-on-your-feet.html, accessed November 8, 2010.

"Nature's expert," Kneipp. https://www.kneipp.com/us_en/natures-expert/water-cure/hydrotherapy/, accessed November 15, 2016.

Shinrin Yoko. http://www.shinrin-yoku.org/shinrin-yoku.html, accessed August 1, 2017.

Websites

www.barebottomshoes.com (Barebottom Shoes)

www.barefootaliance.com (Barefoot Alliance)

www.barefooters.org (Society for Barefoot Living)

www.barefootislegal.com (Barefoot is Legal)

www.barefootprofessor.com (The Barefoot Professor)

www.barefootstrong.com (Dr. Emily Splichal)

www.earthing.com (Earthing)

www.earthinginstitute.net (Earthing Institute)

www.ebfa.com (Evidence-based Fitness Academy)

www.goop.com (Goop)

www.kneipp.com (Kneipping)

www.nutritiousmovement.com (Katy Bowman)

Barefoot is Legal also has an active Facebook Page. Search "Barefoot Is Legal."

Appendix

Foot Anatomy 101 – Biofeedback
Daniel Howell, PhD

Continuing our Foot Anatomy 101 series, I'd like to discuss the role of natural biofeedback to the proper mechanics of walking and running. Natural biofeedback [1] is the gathering of information from body receptors in order to monitor and fine-tune body functions. The brain relies on sensory receptors to gather that information.

There are three types of receptors in the human body: exteroceptors, interoceptors and proprioceptors. Exteroceptors gather information from the outside world; interoceptors gather information from internal organs and proprioceptors keep track of body position. When the brain issues a command to move it receives biofeedback from receptors to ensure that the movement is going as planned. When walking, much of that biofeedback comes from exteroceptors in the soles of the feet. Biofeedback has been underappreciated by podiatrists and foot specialists for decades, but scientists (and runners) are beginning to gain a deeper understanding of its role in human ambulation.

With an estimated 100,000–200,000 exteroceptors in the sole of each foot, your feet are among the most nerve-rich parts of your body. This fact alone should demonstrate the importance of touch to walking and the benefit of going bare for walking properly. But why are there so many nerve endings in the feet? How do those sensitive soles aid walking?

Stand up and walk around (barefoot). When standing and walking, the sole of your foot is the sole part of your body in touch with the environment [2]. Sensory information from the foot is used to protect the foot itself from injury, but it's also used by the brain to make subtle adjustments in your gait to protect bones and joints all the way up your body and to maximize the efficiency of your movements. In others words, it makes walking more fluid and graceful and safe. It takes only milliseconds for sensory information from your foot to reach your brain and for your brain to respond by making adjustments to muscles in your legs, back and arms. By contrast, walking in shoes is far more clumsy and inefficient due (in part) to impaired biofeedback. Muscle contractions, impact forces and joint range-of-motion are measurably different when barefoot [3-8].

Shoe-Induced Neuropathy
A typical walking shoe possesses a hard rubber outer sole and a soft cushioned insole. In addition, people generally wear socks with shoes. These materials lift your feet an inch or more from the ground and silence the biofeedback from exteroceptors. In shoes, the brain receives almost no useful information from the soles of the feet. This lack of sensory feedback is called neuropathy and is considered pathological and dangerous under any other circumstance than shoe-wearing. Because foot biofeedback has been unappreciated for so long, shoe-induced neuropathy has also been ignored by doctors for decades.

Walk Barefoot? On Gravel?
Most people have extremely tender feet after years of wearing shoes.

How to Wear Bare Feet

This tenderness is partly due to the soft and thin skin which has developed from lack of use, but the perception of pain takes place in the brain not the body. Most of us have been told to wear shoes since early childhood; consequently, our brains are unaccustomed to receiving tactile information from the feet. On those rare occasions when we do walk barefoot, our brains receive 'sensory overload' and interpret the strange sensations as painful. Deaf persons who receive their hearing through cochlear implants report their first sounds as painful for the same reason. However, once the brain figures out that the new stimulus is not harmful, the pain subsides. Indeed, what was once considered painful is now re-interpreted as pleasure.

Yes, you can walk and run barefoot on gravel and many other rough surfaces. Gravel poses no threat to your feet, and once your brain discovers this (which can take more than an act of will but time and experience) you can walk on it just fine. And the biofeedback you receive will ensure that your feet and joints are working optimally in addition to providing you with new vistas of pleasure.

Of course, you also need to toughen those tender soles!

****

Footnotes/References:
1. Artificial biofeedback is an attempt to willfully regulate involuntary body functions being externally monitored.
2. The two other nerve-rich body parts—your hands and mouth—are also parts that frequently contact the environment. The use of touch by your hands is obvious, but your mouth must also use touch to monitor what enters your body. Your mouth is sensitive enough to detect an unwanted stray hair in your bite of cheeseburger.

3. Cunningham et al. (2010). The influence of foot posture on the cost of transport in humans. Journal of Experimental Biology 213:790.

4. De Wit et al. (2000). Biomechanical analysis of the stance phase during barefoot and shod running. Journal of Biomechanics 33:269.

5. Wolf et al. (2008). Foot motion in children shoes – a comparison of barefoot walking with shod walking in conventional and flexible shoes. Gait & Posture 27:51.

6. Stacoff et al. (2000). Tibiocalcaneal kinematics of barefoot versus shod running. Journal of Biomechanics 33:1387.

7. Seth (1977). The foot and footwear. Prosthetics and Orthotics International 1:173.

8. Lieberman et al. (2010). Foot strike patterns and collision forces in habitually barefoot versus shod runners. Nature 463:531.

http://barefootprof.blogspot.ca/2011/04/foot-anatomy-101-biofeedback.html

Foot Anatomy 101 – The Special Skin on Your Feet
Daniel Howell, PhD

In this third post in the Foot Anatomy 101 series I'd like to discuss the unique "feetures" of the skin on your feet. Since so much about the feet are unlike other parts of the body, it will probably not surprise you at this point to learn that the skin on your feet is also unique, being especially adapted to the demands of walking and running. Here are some of the special features of 'foot skin': Prints. The skin on the sole of your foot possesses prints. Only the palms of the hands and the soles of the feet possess these tiny undulating folds. The pattern of skin prints on the hands and feet are wholly unique for each person—even genetically identical twins have unique fingerprints and footprints. Your skin prints are also immutable, meaning they do not change over time. For these reasons fingerprints and footprints can be used for identification. But why do we have these prints on our hands and feet? Answer: To improve grip. The prints on your hands help you to grab and hold objects; the prints on your feet increase traction for walking and running. Like the tread on a car tire, those skin folds augment friction to better enable us to grasp the ground and reduce slipping. Unlike car tires which go 'bald' and must be replaced, our skin is self-replenishing, prints and all. Of course, our skin prints are rather useless inside a shoe and many shoe soles are smooth and extremely slippery by comparison, especially under wet conditions.

Sweat Glands
The soles of your feet have a tremendous number of sweat glands. In fact, the three 'sweatiest' parts of your body are your scalp, your

hands and your feet. Although rich in sweat glands, these parts of your body rarely sweat enough to produce dripping sweat; that only occurs under extremely hot conditions or during vigorous exercise. Usually those sweat glands are producing micro-droplets of sweat that quickly evaporate and remove heat from the body. Of course our hands and head are almost always bare and we cover them only under extreme conditions, but our feet are regularly locked away in both shoes and socks. The sweat and heat are thus trapped and the dark, moist, warm, stale conditions inside a shoe become a breeding ground for bacteria and fungi. Shoes are the basic cause of athlete's foot and the best way to avoid or even cure athlete's foot is to go barefoot as much as possible. Enclosing the feet in shoes and socks may also lead to difficulty in regulating body temperature, a condition I call 'hot foot syndrome.'

Attachment
The skin of the sole of the foot is attached to your body exceptionally tightly. The skin on the palms of the hands are similarly attached. You can easily demonstrate this on your hands and feet by pinching the skin. On the top of the foot (and hand) the skin is attached rather loosely to allow flexibility; the skin there can be pinched up and moved about readily. By contrast, the skin of the sole of the foot (and palm of hand) is attached firmly and cannot be easily pinched up or moved side-to-side. This feature increases the skin's resistance to the high sheer forces experienced when walking and running.

These are just four ways the skin on your foot differs from skin on other parts of your body. There are other differences, too, but these four illustrate the point that the feet are remarkably designed for their functions—standing, walking and running. The skin works

How to Wear Bare Feet

best when the foot is bare and kept bare as much as possible. Constantly wearing shoes weakens and softens the skin, making our feet tender and prone to injury. The lack of proper ventilation in closed shoes and socks keeps the skin moist and makes it more vulnerable to invasion by microbes and infection while simultaneously creating the perfect environment for such microorganisms to grow. Going barefoot is healthy for your skin. Calluses and blisters are frequently caused by shoes but rarely result from walking barefoot. With plenty of exposure to sun and air, the skin on your feet will become healthy, strong and beautiful."

http://barefootprof.blogspot.ca/2010/11/special-skin-on-your-feet.html

About the Author

Sue is the author of the best-selling book *My Camino*, which details her journey walking five hundred miles across the north of Spain on an ancient medieval pilgrimage route. Since that first journey, she has returned to the path over twenty times as an expert pilgrim, coaching and guiding groups who want to walk it. Her second book, *Confessions of a Pilgrim*, is about her solo trek on the Portuguese Route carrying a sacred eagle feather. Sue is an internationally acclaimed keynote speaker who has facilitated barefoot and Camino workshops worldwide. As the designer of the first-ever truly barefoot shoe, called Barebottoms, Sue pitched her business idea on the renowned reality show *Dragons' Den*. Her barefoot lifestyle is centered at her lakeside cottage in Canada, and she can often be found walking, running or doing yoga in the forest.

Sue Regan Kenney

Photo credit: Deb Halbot

www.suekenney.ca
www.barebottomshoes.com

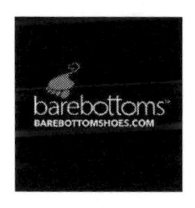

76797983R00066

Made in the USA
Columbia, SC
16 September 2017